The Col

What Are

MW01279881

While it may not be evident, stopped-up plumbing has something to tell us about how to be better patients, painting a boathouse red teaches us how to collaborate to achieve our goals, and hunting for shed deer antlers in early spring offers us practice in commitment. These are among the many life lessons pursued in the parables, allegories, and prose poems of *The Colors of Care*.

This book by Dr. Jerome Freeman is extraordinary in that it deals with the issues of caring not in the form of a treatise, but as a collection of familiar essays. The genre, which had its start with Montaigne, is more like a wayside path than a super-highway. The effort is not to traverse the countryside by the shortest, most direct route, but rather to take a leisurely walk, paying close attention to the surroundings, and to discover along the way some principles by which our lives might be guided.

Dr. Freeman, it is clear from the content of this work, has wandered along many paths; he lives on a large wooded tract along Split Rock Creek in eastern South Dakota, a place crisscrossed with trails into and out of the oaks, along ponds, over bridges, past buildings, across grassy hills. Accompanying him on these walks are friends and relatives who appear often in his accounts, such as his wife Mary; his artist friend Sheila Agee; his son Jason, an aspiring poet; and perhaps most vividly, his father-in-law Francis, a man of uncanny mechanical skill, good common sense, and practical wisdom. Since Dr. Freeman is a practicing physician, a poet, and a teacher of medical ethics, the lessons learned on these sojourns are applicable to the medical profession; they are informed by poetry and are poetic in their own right; and they explore the difficult terrain of medical ethics with convincing authority.

But because Dr. Freeman speaks plainly and directly of matters to which everyone may relate, non-physicians who read the book are afforded an unprecedented glimpse at the way physicians think about their art, how they try to make the right decisions with the patient's health and feelings firmly in mind, and how they struggle with the prickly patches which often get in the way of "doing the right thing." The book will help patients to be better participants in their own care as well as doctors to be better caregivers. Although the essays in the book were originally published in the *South Dakota Journal of Medicine*, the work belongs on the shelves of anyone involved in or interested in thorny medical issues, in the poetry of close observation,\or in the joys and tears encountered in day-to-day living.

The Colors of Care

What Are Those Doctors Thinking?

Other Books by Jerome W. Freeman

The Call to Care
(Ed. and selections, with Arthur Olsen,
Mary Auterman, and Ron Robinson.)
Starting From Here (Poetry)
Easing the Edges (Poetry)
Something at Last (Poetry)
Come and See (Essays)

The Colors of Care

What Are Those Doctors Thinking?

Jerome W. Freeman, M.D.

Ex Machina Publishing Company
Sioux Falls, South Dakota

The cover painting, "Dakota Colors," is an oil on canvas by Sheila Agee of rural Brandon, S.D. Sheila's presence can be discerned in a number of the essays in this book, including "Art and Life."

Published by
Ex Machina Publishing Company
Box 448
Sioux Falls, SD, 57101

Library of Congress Cataloging-in-Publication Data

Freeman, Jerome W.
  The colors of care : what are those doctors thinking? / Jerome W. Freeman.
      p. cm.
  Includes bibliographical references.
  ISBN-13: 978-0-944287-27-9 (pbk.)
  ISBN-10: 0-944287-27-1 (pbk.)
  1. Medical ethics. 2. Medical care. 3. Physician and patient. I. Title.
  R724.F739 2005
  174.2--dc22
                                        2005014326

To Francis
for his inspiration and willingness
to serve as a subject for my reflection; and
to Mary and Jason
for reasons apparent to all who are fortunate enough
to witness their creativity and kindness.

Acknowledgements

This book is published under the auspices of the Center for Ethics and Caring at Sioux Valley Hospital. The author's profits from the sale of *The Colors of Care* are donated back to the Center's publication fund. These funds are used to encourage the publication of works focused on caregiving, ethics and narrative medicine.

The Center for Ethics and Caring is a cooperative effort of Sioux Valley Hospital, Augustana College, the University of South Dakota School of Medicine, and the Good Samaritan Society. The Center provides a variety of resources for those interested in biomedical ethics and caring issues, including professionals in health care, educational institutions, and the community.

The author extends his thanks to Ron and Margaret Robinson for their publishing expertise and to Jennifer Soule, Brad Soule, Ellie Schellinger, and Mary Freeman for their editorial assistance.

Foreword

The essays of this volume appeared in their initial version in the *South Dakota Journal of Medicine* between the years 1996 and 2005. They were written primarily for physicians and other caregivers. The purpose of compiling them here is to promote further discussion of these topics among caregivers and the general public as well. Just as the clinician improves a therapeutic interaction by understanding the patient's narrative, so too an understanding of the clinician's perspective can be helpful to the patient and improve communication between health care provider and patient. Much of the burden of miscommunication seems to reside with the caregiver. But not all of it. Illness care is most effective when the patient is actively working to understand the disease and appreciates the motivation and perspective of the caregiver. Such participation is not always easy and physicians may sometimes seem to actively discourage reciprocal understanding. But it certainly makes sense for anyone with compromised health to have a clear notion of where the caregiver "is coming from."

Obviously, not all physicians perceive ethical quandaries and prioritize goals in the same way. Thus these essays cannot be represented as a definitive explication of every physician's perspective. On the other hand, I believe that the bioethical and psychosocial topics explored in these essays are acknowledged by most physicians to be integral components of medical practice. To that extent, I am hopeful that this text provides an opportunity for the general public to peer into the realm of the caregiver. In these essays, I have tried to honestly reflect upon the motivations, uncertainties and fallibilities that necessarily accompany illness care. Such variables form the context in which health care decisions are made. The titles of these essays are often whimsical and may not clearly define the content. For this reason, the table of contents is annotated, listing the key principles and concepts discussed.

This collection will succeed to the extent that it promotes enhanced understanding and dialogue about illness care. After all, virtually everyone is destined to require some form of medical intervention during the course of a lifetime. All of us should be pondering the query posited in the title of this collection – "What are Those Doctors Thinking?"

JWF

Annotated Table of Contents

Standing By

One summer I spent time "standing by," as it were, while attempts were being made to dig a well on our land. Our initial experience with well drilling, some twenty years earlier, had been fairly uneventful. I assumed that with the second well, a relatively short distance from the first, plentiful water would be found at a similar depth. However, as the well driller sunk the hole deeper and deeper, I began to experience increasing uneasiness with just "standing by" waiting for something to happen. Things were completely beyond my control, and, as it turned out, events proved to be out of the well driller's control, as well. After he had drilled about 500 feet and was preparing to put the drill down one more time preparatory to lowering a pump, the quartzite shifted somewhere below the well casing. Despite multiple attempts, the well driller could not reenter the existing hole that had been so laboriously chiseled out of the quartzite.

As the well driller somberly noted that this experience of hard rock shifting had only happened to him once before, I could not help but make analogies to the idiosyncratic reactions that occur in medicine. Complications of drug therapy and surgery are frequently beyond our control. In acute management of stroke, the "clot buster" TPA can sometimes help dramatically restore a patient. The drama of successful stroke intervention with TPA might be seen as akin to the satisfaction and excitement of finding water when digging a well. And to extend the analogy, discovering that a large cerebral hemorrhage has developed after TPA treatment can be thought of as similiar to the cataclysmic shift of rock that sealed the well driller's hole. In such instances, participants can be left "standing by" helplessly while trying to adjust to events beyond human control.

As I was pondering the above circumstances, another type of "standing by" that is more in our control came to my attention. A friend in another city had a series of vague symptoms that occasioned the need for a MRI. As she recalls this time,

1

she was filled with apprehension about possible bleeding or MS or tumor. Her anxiety continued to build the day after the study as she waited for the result to be called to her. She telephoned her physician at about 9 a.m., leaving word that she was eager to hear the result of the MRI. When she had heard nothing by 4 p.m., she called the office again. She was told that her morning message must have been misplaced and that, in any event, the doctor would not be able to check on the result of the test and give her a report until the following day. Thus, my friend found herself essentially "standing by" for 48 hours as she awaited the result of the test (which ultimately proved to be normal). Perhaps her physician was not overly concerned about the test result and had ordered it as a precaution rather than in the expectation of finding some dire pathology. Nonetheless, for my friend and, I believe, many other patients, the time spent waiting to hear the results of tests can cause great apprehension and dismay.

In this latter type of "standing by," we physicians do have the power to effect remedial action. We can devise office protocols to ensure that patients are rapidly notified of the results of significant tests. There may not always be complete concurrence, of course, in what the physician thinks is important and what the patient deems as critical. However, common sense is a great help. I suspect that most patients are not distressed by waiting several days to receive the results of a routine chemistry panel or perhaps thyroid function testing. On the other hand, it is my experience that most people view any type of brain imaging as a major event. For my friend, 48 hours was too long to wait to be notified that her MRI did not reveal some catastrophic problem. Indeed, this type of circumstance readily lends itself to the wisdom of the golden rule. What physician would wait patiently for two days to learn what his or her own MRI, or one for the physician's family member, revealed? Of course, it is so easy for us, as physicians, to obtain the test results that we almost forget how anxiety provoking just "standing by" can be for patients.

Especially since much can go wrong or is beyond our control in the practice of medicine, physicians should aggressively seize and exploit those opportunities that permit effective intervention. I believe that the timely notification of test results builds good will and confidence on the part of the patient. And obviously we physicians do not need to do this alone. Meaningful teamwork, with appropriate delegation of responsibility to our nursing and clerical staffs, can greatly facilitate this effort.

Of course, there still will be times when both we and our patients need to patiently "stand by" to learn how things will develop. A part of that vigil, we understand, is the inevitability that circumstances will not always turn out as we hope and expect. Physicians need to make a difference where we can. Seeking to ease a patient's burden of expectant waiting is often within our control. We should, to appropriate the title of Saul Bellow's notable novel, "seize the day." In doing so, we will be perceived by our patients and their families as being empathetic and caring. And we will be.

When the Plumbing Failed: An Allegory

In the course of writing and reflection, I generally try to avoid the scatological. It's best that way. However, to paraphrase a vulgar truism, "excrement occurs." And frequently, I might add, at inopportune times.

The day after our family hosted a large social gathering, I was drinking coffee and thinking leisurely morning thoughts. From the bathroom in our bedroom I heard my wife calling urgently to "fling me a nail." At least it sounded like that. Admittedly, I reacted slowly, but eventually I ascertained that she immediately required a pail and dutifully procured one. To my dismay, I learned that our shower had abruptly ceased to drain. The rest of the plumbing seemed secure. Being in a philosophical frame of mind, I sighed "Oh, well," and returned to my coffee. However, when a terse call issued forth a second time, I knew that, to borrow a phrase from Sherlock Holmes, something was afoot. Indeed, now the toilet had ceased to operate, and the water had risen perilously in the stool.

These things always happen, it seems, when one has a houseful of company. Fortunately, one of those visitors was my father-in-law, Francis. Although he is a carpenter and not a plumber, his practical knowledge far surpasses mine. We began a thoughtful analysis of the problem. It seemed that only two drains were malfunctioning – the shower and the stool. We retired to the basement and ascertained that these items were joined at a "y" of large black pipes that then continued onward into unseen depths. Francis, at first, argued for two separate blockages. In his experience, it was not uncommon for multiple systems to fail at the same time. I, on the other hand, used my medical background to argue for a unifying explanation. During a consultative breakfast, I actually drew a sketch of where I postulated the obstruction resided, and Francis conceded some merit to my logic.

At this point, Francis was still hopeful that we might resolve the problem ourselves. I, on the other hand, wanted to enlist the help of a seasoned plumber, preferably a general practice type who could offer an informed analysis of the problem and quickly remedy it. In the old days, when Mary and I had lived in a trailer home, we knew just the person – O'Malley the plumber. O'Malley was known for his colorful expletives and his strong opinions. We had been told that if he did not like a customer on the first visit, he would abruptly leave and never return. Fortunately, he and Mary got along well and O'Malley helped us out of a number of plumbing emergencies. However, he had retired long ago. Thus, I was forced to forego calling the solo practitioner we knew and trusted from the past and, instead, called a large, well-known plumbing contractor. Despite my lyrical descriptions of the urgency of the situation, the scheduler icily informed me that the earliest a plumber could visit our residence was late the next afternoon. I found myself thinking of parallels between my situation and that of a patient calling a physician's office with what is judged to be an important problem. Urgencies, real and perceived, frequently threaten to intrude on the physician's schedule. Sometimes, an effort is made to defer a patient's problem to a time convenient for the office.

Of course, any problem seems most calamitous to the person afflicted. With grim determination, I called a second plumbing outfit. I was told, in what I thought was a somewhat cavalier fashion, that the problem was probably in my septic tank and that this plumbing company would not come out until the septic tank had been pumped.

My demeanor became somber. An easy resolution of the problem did not promise to be forthcoming. When I called the septic tank man, he also told me he couldn't come until the next day. However, within an hour he unexpectedly appeared. I think he actually took pity on me. In any event, he quickly drained the septic tank, seemingly oblivious to the odoriferous aspects of the profession. He proclaimed it to be in good working order and announced that there must be an obstruction in the pipe somewhere in the house, as Francis and I had initially suspected.

5

We were back to where we had started. After offering each other additional thoughts on differential diagnoses, Francis and I visited the first plumbing contractor I had contacted in order to purchase some potent liquid purported to unclog pipes. We were hopeful that this might remedy the problem before the plumber's scheduled visit the next afternoon. However, as we recounted our problem to the shop personnel, we were informed that this liquid process generally doesn't work very well. Furthermore, from our description, they ventured that our difficulty wasn't something their plumbers would work on anyway. What we needed, we were told, is a different kind of specialist – a so-called sewer and drain person. I mused that the equivalent of a gastroenterology consult had been called for.

By now, I admit, I was commencing to feel desperate. I simply wanted the problem fixed. As before, I found myself considering the parallels between my situation and a patient confronting bewildering symptoms. A patient may feel shuffled from one physician to another as a diagnosis is sought. Regrettably, the medical system may seem preoccupied and aloof to such a patient. And, of course, this issue of clogged pipes in one's home is little more than a minor inconvenience as compared to a person confronting a worrisome illness.

The liquid unclogging treatment did not work, as the retailer had predicted. With trepidation, I placed still another call – this time to the sewer and drain company. To my surprise they were personable and willing to respond quickly. The company technician was at our doorstep within an hour, armed with a menacing array of coiled pipe that terminated in a knife-like mechanism. His diagnostic appraisal was precise and to the point. After pounding on various pipes in our basement, he announced that most likely the obstruction was in the black drain pipe as it traversed the foundation and headed for the septic tank. When questioned as to why he thought the problem was in that location (since not all of the drains in the house seemed to be affected), he didn't choose to elaborate much beyond his conviction that he understood the problem. Fortunately, he was right.

Again, parallels exist with medicine. Certainly, there are times when I see a patient and a lengthy differential diagnosis can be generated. However, based on the nuances of a patient's history and my examination, I generally have a good instinct as to the ultimate etiology of the problem. This is true for most physicians, I suspect.

Sometimes one may succeed in extending clinical experience to nonmedical realms of life. I did develop a plausible differential diagnosis as to the site of my plumbing difficulties. However, in the end, I needed to defer to the more definitive expertise of someone in that field. In many walks of life, rote knowledge may be very helpful, but not sufficient. Wisdom and experience must also be applied. On this subject, most plumbers and physicians would agree.

Art and Life

Sheila paints the sky over and over again. Sometimes she uses a single canvas. At other times multiple panels, such as a sky triptych, are linked together. Every sky is unique. Her paintings help me appreciate the varied hues that surround us. Gradations of blue may be layered upon one another, while yellows and grays are subtly blended with secondary colors.

And clouds, of course, appear frequently. They may reflect the auburn of a setting sun or be the harbinger of an approaching storm. Some towering clouds may suggest a virtually palpable texture, while others are such faint whispers as to require a second look to verify their presence.

Often, after studying Sheila's paintings, I gaze at the sky around me. On occasional days it seems sensual and intimate, at other times, aloof. Twice, recently, I have actually called Sheila to alert her to spectacular evening colors. Having become a better observer, I assume the role of a sky expert. I'm bemused, intrigued, or awed depending on the hour and the day. It is fascinating to move from a canvas to the sky and back again. Invariably, both nature and Sheila's art have it right.

There is some evidence that systematically exposing medical students to works of art enhances their clinical powers of observation. At Yale, all first year medical students take an "art-in-medicine" course. The students are encouraged to analyze works of art, making observations and deductions. Irwin Braverman, the professor who coordinates the class, has data to indicate that his students' diagnostic skills were 50% better than students not enrolled in the class.[1]

Visual arts can function, I suppose, like narrative forms. We learn from the stories we tell one another. Certainly, this is true in patient care. How well we do as clinicians is frequently dependent on how carefully we listen to the content of the history and to the emotions that attend it. Literary narratives – novels, short stories, and poetry – can also offer abundant insight into the human condition. As we immerse ourselves in stories, we are exposed to a wide range of motivations, dilemmas, and possible responses. Sometimes the characters of fiction are noble and inspiring, while at other times they may be nefarious. Regardless, well done narrative insistently engages us. And the Yale experience suggests that the study of visual arts can similarly broaden our understanding of the human condition.

When my nephew, Justin, was about four years old, he began to refer to Sheila, the artist, as "Aunt Sheila." From Justin's perspective at that time, all women of a certain age (*i.e.*, the age of my wife and her sisters) were aunts. At some point, as Justin grew older, his perspective enlarged, and he gained the ability to distinguish the difference between a good friend and biologic family. In a fashion somewhat analogous to Justin's process of maturation, a caregiver's perceptions and understanding can gain sophistication by a focused attention upon the complexities of people's lives and the influences that surround them. How we view things depends on our perspective or, as philosopher William F. May says, "our angle of vision."[2]

We can never know enough. While I might instinctively appreciate a painting, an art expert like Sheila can invariably enrich my understanding by her analysis. In addition to explaining technique, she situates artist and the art in a cultural context. She delves into the meaning of things. Similarly, the search for meaning is really what clinicians do when we analyze a patient's historical narrative. Art and life have layers of significance, some readily discernable and others obscure and concealed. Sometimes the statement is made that society should appreciate "art for art's sake." More to the point, we should cherish art for our sake. Visual art, like narrative, can teach us about ourselves and those we serve. In so doing, it enhances our capacity as caregivers.

**Sheila Agee is an artist who lives and does her creative work in rural Brandon. Her paintings have periodically appeared as covers on the South Dakota Journal of Medicine.

References
[1] USA Weekend, December 28-30, 2001.
[2] May WF. The Patient's Ordeal. Indiana University Press; 1991.

Truth and Memory

"How is it possible to bring order out of memory?" With this query Beryl Markham begins her famous memoir, *West With the Night*.[1]

Markham's question prompts me to recall Memory Lodge, an idyllic sounding place my wife's family has talked about for years. The trail of this collective memory began in 1965. My father-in-law, Francis, took his wife and four children on an extended vacation highlighted by a stop at the World's Fair in New York. The leisurely trip home took them across Canada and somewhere north of Thunder Bay they discovered Memory Lodge. Their time at the Lodge must have been a splendid finale to their trip. Francis and his children enthusiastically recalled open fields with flowers, exciting woodlands, and an enchanting stream.

One summer, some twenty-five years after their initial visit to Memory Lodge, I proposed that the family reassemble there. All agreed that this was one of my better ideas, and excitement for the return visit steadily grew. Even the in-laws were enthusiastic. The youngest children, not yet born when the original trip was made, seemed pleased that they too would finally be able to claim part of this family legacy of Memory Lodge.

On the appointed day our caravan of vehicles left Grand Marais, Minnesota, and headed north. With the great Lake Superior on our right and towering, wooded hills on our left, we eagerly proceeded to the Canadian border and beyond. Although the scenery was marvelous, we all anticipated that it was a mere prelude to the satisfactions that awaited our arrival at the Lodge.

When we finally came upon a dilapidated sign proclaiming the entrance to Memory Lodge, I recall a sense of collective puzzlement beginning to develop in our group. What we encountered seemed vastly different from the family memory and lore of Memory Lodge. Actually, there was no "lodge" as such, but rather several ramshackle buildings resembling an

11

old motel. On their perimeter, a sluggish trickle of water wended its discouraged way along a gully. Periodic scattered trees and bushes stood in the background but no lush forest was visible.

Gravely, we emerged from our cars and looked for the proprietor. Several of the rental units had doors ajar, and we peeked in to get a sense of the accommodations. Each room had faded linoleum, discolored wallpaper, and beds seeming to sag from the burden of many seasonal visitors. As our group gathered about outside one of the rooms, the manager emerged to make our acquaintance. She seemed surprised that we had actually arrived, despite the fact that we had made reservations many weeks earlier. She also apologetically explained that our rooms would not all be adjoining, as we had requested, because a large church youth group had extended their stay and was using some of the rooms that had been intended for us.

At this point, by consensus, we acknowledged a startling disparity between this aging resort and fond memories the family held of a visit here twenty-five years earlier. The manager seemed to agree with our verdict that we should not even check in. Clearly, she was preoccupied with the rowdy youth group. Somewhat sheepishly our family members returned to Thunder Bay. But that night we thoroughly enjoyed reminiscing about both sets of experiences of Memory Lodge—those created by a young family in 1965 and those of our rueful return visit.

As I was reflecting upon the interplay of memory and contemporary reality, I recalled one of my college texts that dealt with the issue of homecoming. The author stressed that one's experiences and inevitable maturity ensure that the home place of memory can never be truly recaptured. While obvious elements from one's younger days may persist, the reality of a homecoming is inevitably changed by new perspectives. My recall of this thesis seemed so relevant to reflections on memory that I actually spent some time paging through various old philosophy and literature books from my college years, hoping to find the original source. I didn't succeed, and it is probably just as well. Very likely, the misplaced book wasn't as eloquent and pithy as my memory suggested.

One can move quite readily from the nostalgia of family memories and college enthusiasms to the disquiet many people have when comparing today's medical practice with the "old days." The public remembers kindly general practitioners and house calls. Practicing physicians recall a time when DRGs did not force premature hospital discharges and insurance companies did not require tedious pre-certifications. But of course one can no more return to the old days of medicine than our family was able to recapture the magic of the first visit to Memory Lodge. Life and circumstances irrevocably change. And as a good aspect of that transformation, health care providers enjoy unprecedented capabilities. If, professionally, we truly were somehow thrown back into a former practice era, it would be most disquieting.

Arguably, our professional challenge is to flourish in the modern realm of health care while honoring the memories and traditions of the past. Our clinical abilities can be enriched by memory without requiring us to flounder in a quagmire of wistful reminiscences. My family has fond memories of Memory Lodge and the two trips that were made there. But none of us wish to return!

References

[1] Markham B. West With the Night. New York: Northpoint Press; 1942, 1983.

Improbable Lives

My wife and I met our friends in Omaha. The principle reason for our visit was to view the Andrew Wyeth Exhibition at the Joselyn Art Museum. His entire "Helga series" of paintings was on display. We learned that Wyeth kept this collection secret during the 14 years he painted Helga. We all found it fascinating to imagine the collaboration between Wyeth and Helga and to witness her visual transformation into middle age over the course of their association.

The afterglow of these magnificent paintings suffused about us as we departed the museum in search of our cars. But our mood was bitterly disrupted when our friends discovered that their car had been vandalized in broad daylight. The passenger window was shattered and a purse stolen.

In the aftermath of regret and recrimination, a certain irony interposed itself into my reflections. Several weeks earlier, this aggrieved couple and we had joined eight others on a whirlwind journey through Paris and northern Italy. We had been warned repeatedly of pickpockets and other forms of theft and throughout our journey judiciously guarded our wallets and purses. No untoward incidents occurred during this European sojourn. Now we all found it disquieting to be visiting a local community and to experience the very type of crime we had so feared and worked to avoid in Europe.

The juxtaposition of these two trips — one to Europe and the other to neighboring Omaha — is not meant to be overly profound. It seems however to reinforce the obvious. Life is a puzzlement and often unpredictable.

Some years ago I cared for a middle-aged woman who had spent most of her adult life working to stay healthy. She ate no meat, jogged daily, and espoused regular yoga. Her reaction to my reluctant revelation that she had a brain tumor was one of utter disbelief. It seemed impossible to her that someone who had lived in such a healthy fashion as she could develop a malignant cancer. In the days and weeks that followed she would repeatedly ask how this could possibly have happened

14

to someone who strived to maintain healthy habits. I could only agree with her that her situation was a tragic quandary.

Another patient also comes to mind. He, too, was middle-aged and seemingly healthy. A month before I met him, he struck his head forcefully on an overhead object at his place of employment. When he learned from me that his subsequent headaches were not from the blow, but were in fact a brain tumor, he and his wife were insistent that the head injury must have caused the tumor. To their way of thinking, it was obvious. He had been in perfect health until he struck his head. He then developed headaches, and the tumor was discovered. Surely, they argued, there had to be a causal relationship between his recent head trauma and the brain tumor. My gentle attempt to disabuse them of this belief over the weeks that followed met with little success. I believe this couple thought I was somehow working to protect his employer from a workers' compensation action.

The world is filled with the improbable, giving lie to our naïve beliefs that we generally control our destinies and can explain the circumstances that surround us. Some weeks after our group of European travelers returned, my office staff received an unusual telephone call. Jasmine, an employee in a neighboring medical office, inquired if I had recently been in Europe. She had been admiring photographs her cousin had brought back from his own trip to Europe, and she thought she recognized me in one of them. Sure enough, she brought to my office a photo of me standing next to her cousin in front of the Mona Lisa. Certainly, I did not know him or realize, at the time, that he was from South Dakota. The likelihood is astonishingly small that anyone would be coincidentally captured in a photograph in front of the world's most famous painting and then have that photograph find its way into the hands of an acquaintance in one's hometown. Most of us look at such travel photographs superficially. I am still amazed that Jasmine looked at the photograph closely enough to recognize me and then contacted my office. Presumably, it is the same type of amazing serendipity that results in some people winning a lottery jackpot. The odds are prohibitively arrayed against such occurrences.

More and more, it seems, when I talk to patients and families, I find myself using the phrase "it's out of our hands." I must ruefully acknowledge that there is much I can't predict in terms of why diseases occur and what the clinical course will be. Even in the case of a malignant brain tumor, I am unable to specifically predict how long a person will survive or the precise circumstances that will surround the ultimate demise.

In some respects, I was more sure of answers at the beginning of my career than I am now. More and more I sense the imponderable insinuating itself into ordinary lives. Sometimes when I am with medical students, especially in their initial preclinical years, I am amused at how certain they are of what they know. Many of my associates have made similar observations. Recently, a colleague of mine was discussing psychosocial issues with some first year medical students. One student impatiently raised his hand to point out that most of the class was not destined to become psychiatrists and therefore the topic at hand was irrelevant to them. From the vantage point of extensive clinical experience, such a comment seems utterly naïve and unfounded. But in truth, none of us can fully appreciate what we don't know. What can differentiate innocence and experience is the ability to suspend one's instinctive convictions that life should be logical and predictable. Certainly in the care of patients, where idiosyncrasies abound, caregivers need to respect the improbable and the unplanned for. Much is beyond human control. Surprises, good and bad, are lurking everywhere.

The Future Past

On a recent trip to central Minnesota, my wife read aloud Anton Chekhov's short story "Gooseberries." At one point, the protagonist makes the haunting observation:

> "There ought to be behind the door of every happy, contented man someone standing with a hammer continually reminding him with a tap that there are unhappy people; that however happy he may be, life will show him her laws sooner or later, trouble will come for him-disease, poverty, losses, and no one will see or hear, just as now he neither sees nor hears others."[1]

These words necessarily focus us upon what we possess and what we've lost or may lose. While Chekhov is anticipating a still opaque future, his sentiments could also pertain to the events and relationships of a previous time.

I continued to think of Chekhov's admonitions during the rest of the day, pondering the future and the past. As it happened, that afternoon I had the opportunity to visit with a 78 year old woman who, in her youth, had known my father. Indeed, to put the matter more accurately, they had been sweethearts. In the years before his death, my father had fondly mentioned Betty from time to time. And as I visited with her, it was clear that Betty still remembered my father with great affection. At one point during our visit, she hesitantly produced a photograph of herself, taken at age 19. She had dressed for a friend's wedding, and, quite simply, she was stunning. She recalled taking the train all the way to Chicago to visit my father, who was attending Rush Medical School. Her husband was present, and she acknowledged that he had never heard these recollections before but he seemed undisturbed by the account of the adventure. As we sat around her kitchen table, Betty shyly produced a sterling silver necklace

17

and bracelet, a set that my father had once given to her as a gift. Betty wanted my wife to have this jewelry since she herself did not have a daughter.

I'm not sure at what point in their young lives my father and Betty parted ways. Betty explained that they bowed to the proscriptions of that day against interfaith marriages. Some 60 years after that difficult decision, she sounded wistful. One had the idea that there was still some yearning for what might have been.

As my wife and I drove away from their home, I found myself railing against the strictures and customs of a society that in one age can cause deep anguish and then, in the next generation, be essentially discarded. My wife did point out that I should not grieve the course of history too much, in this case. If Betty and my father had abjured their families' religious beliefs and married, that certainly would have precluded my existence. I believe at that point in our conversation I changed the subject.

Presumably, Chekhov's reflections on life and loss were enriched by the fact that he was a physician, as well as a writer. While medicine obviously does not lend an exclusive truth to writing, it can, at times, reveal the essence of human experience. Through his protagonist's voice, Chekhov may well have been recounting truths learned from medical practice. Indeed, I would venture to say that virtually all physicians find themselves sharing, to some degree, the burdens of their patients—a career devastated by a bad business decision, a love squandered, or health and vigor lost.

It is tempting to imagine a world free of suffering and illness. Of course, such a place would not be our world. While tempted to bemoan what has or will befall us, I am reminded of Robert Frost's reflections in his poem "Birches" as he dreamed of climbing a birch tree toward Heaven: "Earth's the right place for love, I don't know where it's likely to go better."[2]

All of life is adaptation. In a sense, what we do in medicine largely involves helping people accommodate to change and inevitability. In this process, we can be sustained by our dreams of what might be in the future, or could have been in the past. Betty and my father were not necessarily unique in their love and their loss. As I think about their lives 60 years ago and the people I'm privileged to know and help care for today, I come back again to the truth of Frost's observation about our world being the "right place for love." We are defined by our loves and our losses.

References

[1] Chekhov A. Gooseberries. In: Hansen R, Shephard J, editors. You've Got to Read This. Perennial; 2000.
[2] Frost R. The Poetry of Robert Frost. Lathem EC, editor. New York: Holt, Rinehart and Winston; 1969.

To Redeem One Person...

In today's society, many people yearn for more quiet time. There is talk of the need to step back and reflect. Often, however, it seems that the urgencies of our lives interfere. Sometimes I find that leisurely reflection is deferred until I suspend various commitments by leaving town.

Recently, my wife and I traveled to Minneapolis with two friends. On our first evening there, we were joined for dinner by a Minneapolis couple not well known to our Sioux Falls friends. The six of us had an animated conversation throughout the evening. Afterwards, Mary and I commented to each other about how gracious and engaging the Minneapolis couple was to our other friends. We had observed this social skill on earlier occasions as well. This couple invariably seeks out new individuals and earnestly visits with them.

The following morning at breakfast, Mary and I complimented the couple on how interested and committed they seem in such social settings. To our surprise, they indicated that this behavior was very conscious and deliberate on their part. They went on to explain that when they first moved to Minneapolis his company had hosted a reception for them. At the preliminary social hour, company executives and spouses had come over to meet the new couple. However, when it was time for the meal, the other executives and their companions seemed to quickly disperse, seeking seating with familiar individuals. The new couple, our friends, were literally left standing alone trying to decide how to inconspicuously find a place to sit. Both of them felt abandoned. They had the perception of being superficially welcomed and then left to fend for themselves. As a result of that experience, this couple explicitly decided to help others, whom they might meet in the future, from being subjected to similar feelings of isolation. As evidenced at our dinner meeting in Minneapolis, their efforts are effective and appreciated.

As I reflected on this subject, I recalled a poem I wrote several years ago that comments on the superficiality and posturing that can sometimes take place in social situations:

> At the reception
> we stand nervously
> near one another
> reciting pleasantries
> and plotting how
> to graciously excuse
> ourselves for a move
> toward brighter stars
> in the social galaxy.

Throughout the remainder of that weekend in Minneapolis, I found myself thinking about our friends' commitment to being interested in whomever they meet. As can sometimes happen with reflection, I proceeded to make related associations. A member of our group praised Caroline Kennedy's new anthology of the poetry cherished by her mother, Jacqueline Kennedy Onassis. On the basis of this recommendation, I promptly purchased the book. One poem I found particularly moving was "Ithaca" by Constantine P. Cavafy.[1] Cavafy, in effect, talks about the importance of relishing our daily experiences in life rather than merely focusing on future goals that may prove illusive and unobtainable. He uses Ithaca as a metaphor for the objectives we may set for ourselves. Cavafy's poem includes the following stanzas:

> When you set out on your journey to Ithaca,
> pray that the road is long,
> full of adventure, full of knowledge . . .
> Always keep Ithaca in your mind.
> To arrive there is your ultimate goal.
> But do not hurry the voyage at all.
> It is better to let it last for many years;
> and to anchor at the island when you are old,
> rich with all you have gained on the way . . .

21

By analogy, we all have our "Ithacas." We may be focused on our jobs, our families, financial concerns, or prospects for leisure. Cavafy's poem, just like the efforts of our friends to actively engage whomever they encounter in social situations, speaks to the importance of not overlooking people in our hurried effort to reach anticipated ends. Indeed, the most precious aspects of our days may often be the unanticipated event or accidental encounter.

Still another literary connection to my weekend reflections presented itself. Someone casually mentioned the book *To Redeem One Person is to Redeem the World*. This is a biography of the famed psychotherapist Frieda Fromm-Reichmann. I found myself repeatedly thinking about this title and its possible implications for the healing professions. After returning home from our trip, I was able to secure a copy. In the prologue, the author, Gail Hornstein, mentions a great sixteenth-century rabbi, Isaac Luria, who noted: "A divine spark is attached to each prayer, each charitable act, each moment of goodness . . . To assist another is to do God's work. To redeem one person is to redeem the world."[2] In adopting this latter phrase as the title of her biography, Hornstein emphasizes the power of commitment. Put simply, each person has the ability to nourish and enrich the lives of others.

When we are most successful in medicine, the patient feels "first in importance." This can occur when the clinician earnestly seeks to understand the patient's personal narrative. In so doing, the clinician gains insight into contextual influences. The merits of such dedicated attention are implicitly championed in the poem "Ithaca." Clearly, such an emphasis is also evident in the stirring challenge of "redeeming the world" by one's dedication to the welfare of another person. And such intent characterizes the Minneapolis couple who resolutely champions and nourishes each opportunity to interact with new acquaintances.

In medicine we attend to specifics. What is needed, perhaps, is the courage to cast aside those distractions that might otherwise distort our focus. This is not to discount the appeal of an idealized "Ithaca" shimmering on some distant horizon. But more immediate concerns rise up before us. Our patients are at hand.

References

[1] Cavafy CP. Ithaca. In: Kennedy C, editor. The Best Loved Poems of Jacqueline Kennedy Onassis. New York: Hyperion; 2001.
[2] Hornstein GA. To Redeem One Person is to Redeem the World. New York: The Free Press; 2000.

Fence Dreams

Twenty-five years ago, when I returned to South Dakota with my family to begin practice, we chose to live in the country and have never regretted it. All persons are influenced by their environment, and, periodically, I am struck by the notion that living outside of town necessarily shapes one's perspectives on certain issues. Take for instance one's view of walls and fences. In town, fences generally are constructed to protect privacy or as decorative additions. More practical functions are paramount in the country. Typically, one must remain vigilant for any breach in a fence's integrity. Regular fence repair must be performed in order to keep livestock in or out, depending on one's commitments.

When doing the annual work of fence repair, I invariably think of Frost's poem, "Mending Wall."[1] I recall the beginning of the poem, "Something there is that doesn't love a wall..." and remember the repeated adage, "Good fences make good neighbors." This spring was no exception to such reflection. Especially since my neighbors to the north and south are no longer grazing cattle, I had to legitimately query "what I was walling in or walling out and to whom I was likely to give offense" as I went about the repair of the barbed wire.

A fence need not be performing a specific duty in order to justify maintaining it. Frost portrays companionable neighbors doing fence work as part of a spring ritual. There is something to be said for demarcating one's space. In the country, it is customary to survey the neighbor's land from the vantage point of one's own territory, and, of course, neighbors can readily visit each other across the fence. On suitable occasions it's an easy matter for adjacent landowners to go over, or through, the type of country fence I'm extolling.

In addition to mending fence this spring, I also undertook a project to remove sections of old, neglected barbed wire. This is always a tedious job and fraught with some danger as one battles the unexpected recoil of ancient wire. The best way to accomplish the task is slowly and methodically. As I worked, I imagined the fencers who preceded. The rust on the barbed wire and the old hardware suggested that portions of the fence had been there for many decades. Sometimes lengths of wire had been carefully mended with secure splices. In other places, strands of barbed wire were more haphazardly joined by connecting loops. Sections of fence that had been sturdily effective in earlier times were now collapsed and lying partially buried in the soil. Metal t-posts, once carefully aligned by my unknown predecessors, were now bent askew, while the occasional wooden post displayed the crevices of fracture and decay.

Invariably, it seems, such ancient fences wandered off the survey lines, at least as they are determined today. Perhaps approximation was culturally more acceptable in the olden days. Besides, it was easier to go around large obstacles such as trees and rocks rather than trying to transect them. Modern day evidence of how early settlers "made do" is occasionally discovered in gnarled boxelder trees that contain pieces of barbed wire grown into their trunks.

As I immersed myself in the ceremony of this year's fencing, I pondered human lives and motivation. We want to secure what seems our own. We yearn for the predictable and true. Who among us would not choose to protectively fence our lives and those of our loved ones from the turmoil and tragedy of the outside world? Who, if given the chance, would not readily opt to erect a barrier to thwart illness and death?

Of course our instincts to metaphorically fence ourselves off from tragedy and dismay are an understandable response to the human condition. While we long for our lives to be linear and predictable like a well-constructed fence, we cannot ordinarily avoid disappointments and disruptions. Perhaps this adds to the appeal of fencing. As one ratchets the stretcher to make barbed wire taut and deftly twists post clips to render it secure, one enjoys the illusion that things can be made right in the world. Sometimes reassurances, even if illusory, are helpful. This can be true for patients and their caregivers alike. In times of such respite, we catch our breath and prepare to reenter the fray.

References
[1] Frost R. Mending Wall. In: Latham EC, editor. The Poetry of Robert Frost. New York: Holt, Rinehart & Winston; 1969.

Shifting Gears

My brother had a treasured '58 Ford pickup that he reluctantly sold to me when he moved to New York. For a number of years, I used it for plowing snow in the winter and periodically visiting the county dump. I recalled that truck recently while visiting with friends about embarrassing episodes we had each experienced.

On one memorable occasion, I was joined in the cramped cab of the pickup by my sister, who was visiting from Washington, DC. She had become more sophisticated while living out East, and I detected an element of unspoken disdain when she climbed into the truck. However, I assured her that the trips to the dump were almost invariably exciting. Although the junk and debris piled into the back generally did not fall out (at least to my knowledge), it usually looked like it was about to. This trip was no exception, and I was eager to reach our destination and unload the cargo.

As I waited at a stop sign to enter a main thoroughfare, I recall being surprised at the volume of traffic. Finally, my impatience exceeded my prudence, and I lurched forward between two cars. The faulty clutch in the truck made such abrupt starts somewhat perilous, and the balky steering wheel demanded close concentration to avoid overcompensation. As I tried to valiantly pick up speed to match the cars I had joined, I reflexively glanced in the rearview mirror. This was a largely futile gesture since my cargo covered the rear window. Stoically, I peered through the cracked side mirror that clung to my door. At that point, it dawned on me that the cars behind, like those ahead, all had their headlights on. Inadvertently, I had burst into the middle of a funeral procession.

I curbed my natural instinct to abruptly swing out of line. This was probably fortunate because swerving vigorously would have unsettled my cargo and complicated my difficulties. Rather, I calmly decided that my best option was to signal my intention to leave the procession, especially since the car behind me was following very closely. Unfortunately, the truck's turn signals had been inoperative for some time, and manual signaling from the truck was always compromised by the difficulty of rolling down the driver's window while still trying to steer and shift gears.

As I struggled with these maneuvers, my sister slumped down in her seat and pulled her hat over her face. This was not the type of intrepid demeanor I had anticipated from a resident of our nation's capitol. I tried to make light commentary to bolster her spirits, pointing out that the mourners probably had more weighty things on their minds than our unsightly truck thrust into their midst. She did not seem to cheer up much. Finally, with the side window partially down, I was able to signal a right turn and cautiously downshift, before exiting onto a side street. No one, as far as I could tell, honked or gestured at us as we crept away. All in all, I believe I recovered from the trauma of this embarrassing incident more quickly than my sister. I have since noted that she still blanches at the mention of that day.

Often our life experiences mirror those in medical practice. On occasion, I have endured somewhat comparable embarrassments and indignities in the course of patient care. Indeed recently, when I was running behind in my schedule, I rushed into a room to see a patient with Parkinson's disease. A husband and wife were sitting there patiently waiting for me. I pulled up my stool in front of the husband and began to question how he was feeling. After a brief pause, his wife timidly observed that she was the one with Parkinson's, not her husband. As one might imagine, I was most embarrassed. If I had recalled the funeral procession incident, as I sat with this couple, I might have been prompted to invoke Yogi Berra's observation that this seemed "like déjà vu all over again." I clearly had to metaphorically shift gears and extricate myself from this blunder. While not recalling all of the details, I do know that I told the woman (truthfully) that my mistake was a fortuitous one. Her Parkinson's medications were working so well she really did not have any obvious features of the disease. After the couple left, however, I began to worry about what the

28

husband would think when he awoke during the night wondering why, if his wife looked so good, I had assumed he was the one with Parkinson's.

Clearly it is helpful for a physician to think quickly and to be willing to reevaluate. Over time, I have learned that if a patient or family suggests a patently unlikely diagnosis, it should not be summarily rejected out of hand. On occasion, they are right. It is more prudent to sagely nod when unlikely conjectures are made, rather than later trying to reconcile why one's working differential did not include the correct diagnosis. Some years ago, for instance, I evaluated a young woman who was certain that she had multiple sclerosis. Her demeanor and lack of objective physical findings on examination made me convinced she had a somatoform disorder. Fortunately, I did obtain a MRI of her head. It revealed the classic lesions of MS. Then, suddenly, her myriad of ill-defined complaints made sense. Her symptoms had not changed but my perception of them certainly had.

One thing that I have learned and relearned in practice is the importance of acknowledging my blunders and retreating from them as quickly as possible, much like my sheepish exit from the funeral procession. Of course one's clinical mistakes cannot always be rectified. When we are afforded the opportunity to extricate ourselves from peril, we should humbly accept it and move on.

Being There

The office nurse and I moved rapidly down the hospital corridor. We still had several patients to see before starting in the clinic. The day seemed to portend many obligations and insufficient time.

My companion had become an office nurse some 20 years earlier by virtue of having left full-time hospital work to join a physician practice. Even though she frequently participated in hospital rounds, she was still assigned an "office" designation in the eyes of the hospital staff. By implication, perhaps, she had escaped the rough and tumble world of acutely ill patients and, in so doing, abdicated the skills needed in that setting.

One of the patients whose room we darted into had been struggling with progressive liver failure. We arrived at a time of crisis. Carter had just rushed into the bathroom to have a bowel movement and sat down upon the toilet without lifting the lid. Having been hastily bathed by the hospital staff, Carter was now sitting on the edge of his bed and adamantly refusing to get into the wheelchair to go to the radiology department. The office nurse, who had known Carter for some time, stepped past me and the two aides who were warily considering his new intransigence. Putting her hand on his arm, she patiently explained to him why it was important to have his x-ray done. Carter nodded reluctantly and asked her if she'd help him put his underpants on. "You won't be embarrassed, will you?" he asked shyly. She deftly slipped his shorts over his swollen legs and then stood closely by so that he could lean against her as she pulled the shorts all the way up.

Carter then sat down again firmly on the edge of the bed. "I need to wash my hands first," he declared. Acting as if she had all morning (while I furtively glanced at my watch and thought of patients waiting at the clinic), the office nurse filled the shallow basin with warm water and added a bar of soap. She moved over to Carter and gently washed his hands while he gazed at her solemnly. He seemed to bask in her attention as

30

she assisted his languid ablutions. She then carefully dried his hands before expertly assisting his wobbly effort to stand, pivot, and drop into the wheelchair. The aides and I were so mesmerized by the solemnity and innocence of this communion, that none of us even moved forward to assist the transfer.

On that day, she was just being a nurse, I suppose. She is always a nurse when summoned to care. Seemingly without forethought, she intervened to do what was needed to comfort Carter. Watching her, it seemed clear to me that the most noble things we caregivers do frequently are the types of humble, compassionate actions I was observing.

As I reflect back upon this episode, I remain subdued by its lessons. Whether caring for the patient as a nurse, a therapist, or a physician, some things should be at the heart of what we do. A gentle touch, undistracted presence, and soothing communication all have enduring value.

Clearly the physician has a complex role that includes orchestrating diagnosis and therapy. But for the patient, there are times when such cerebral talents are simply not enough. On such occasions, the patient is not asking for more than we can give, but for what we may not think to offer. By attending to particulars, by recalling stellar examples of caregiving previously encountered, the physician can excel at the gentle art of comforting. This should be our mandate whether we have the concomitant ability to offer curative treatment or not. It's the reason for being there.

Courtesy

We were leaving Orange County after a family wedding. During our several day visit, the weather had been spectacular. On the morning of our scheduled departure, however, dense fog rolled in. The passengers throughout the terminal could be overheard speculating on whether their flights would be able to take off. In the end, our flight was only delayed by 30 minutes. As the plane neared the Denver Airport it was apparent that many of my fellow passengers were apprehensive about being able to meet their connecting flights. Certainly we were. It began to appear that we had, at best, fifteen minutes to exit our plane and find the new gate. When our plane was in the landing process, and again while it was taxiing to the gate, the flight attendants used the intercom to stress the fact that a number of passengers had very tight flight connections. They requested that when the plane's door was opened, all passengers not faced with a dire time crunch remain seated to allow others to exit rapidly. But when the plane stopped, virtually every passenger ahead of us stood up to join the waiting queue. Our escape from the plane was frustratingly slow.

It seemed to me quite certain that many of the people ahead of us did not have a desperately close flight connection. Rather, they were simply eager to exit the plane and get on with their morning activities. Perhaps, because I was so personally affected by the prospect of missing our connecting flight, I was struck by the selfishness of these actions. I knew that if we missed our flight, we probably would be delayed in the Denver airport for six hours or so until another scheduled flight departed. I hated the idea. As I waited for the many people ahead of me to exit the plane, I fumed at what I perceived to be the lack of common courtesy and decency in our society.

Shortly after this California visit, I was passing an emergency room and was stopped by a surgeon. He was extremely unhappy and wanted to talk at some length about the indignities he sustained at the hands of physician colleagues who neglect common courtesies. A patient with symptomatic gallstones had been sent to the emergency room with the instruction that he be seen by this surgeon. The referring physician had not called the surgeon to say that the patient was coming. Nor had any records been sent. The surgeon was particularly angry because he felt that this problem would have best been handled by a routine office visit leading to a scheduled surgery. I think what upset this physician was his perception that professional collegiality and common courtesy are frequently neglected in health care. He went on to cite several other examples. Often, when consulted to see a critically ill patient in the hospital, he recalled receiving the message from a ward secretary rather than from the referring physician. The surgeon felt that a personal call from the primary physician would lead to much better patient care. It would enable the surgeon to know the severity of the patient's problem and to better judge how quickly the patient should be seen. Another example the surgeon cited was the common request that a hospital consult be seen on an emergency basis even when the patient's problem was not urgent and could easily be handled in a more routine fashion.

There is, I think, truth in this surgeon's observations that we physicians do not always treat each other with appropriate collegiality and consideration. Multiple examples might be summoned to support this contention. We have all known instances in which a physician is unnecessarily critical of the work of another caregiver. And surely there are occasions in which physicians' only communication with each other, as they care for the same patient, is a cursory note in the hospital chart. Occasionally the written order of one physician is summarily changed by another without these physicians otherwise communicating. Especially when physicians are busy and preoccupied, medical care can fall into patterns that do not promote teamwork and mutual regard, nor the best interest of the patient.

But I have strayed from my opening anecdote. My family and I did make our plane connection in Denver. It was close. After a seemingly interminable wait to get off the first plane, we discovered that we had to get from concourse B to concourse A in order to catch our flight. This involved racing down a long flight of stairs, waiting for an electric train to take us to the "A" building, and then racing up another long flight of stairs to reach the main floor. As we approached the gate, with our luggage in tow, the waiting area seemed deserted. I could still see the plane at the ramp, but it seemed futile to gesticulate from the window or throw myself on the floor in abject frustration. Suddenly a phone rang, and from around a barrier a single airline employee emerged to answer it. She was being alerted that we were on our way. She in turn called the airplane, the ramp was reopened, and we were ushered to our seats. And if that wasn't enough, the flight was smooth and arrived in Sioux Falls precisely on time.

Even though some of my fellow passengers had seemed rude and inconsiderate earlier, the airline personnel were consistently courteous during the ordeal that morning. It seems that it would have been quite easy for the airline staff to have authorized our flight to leave before we arrived at the gate. Indeed I can recall at least one time in the past when I arrived at the gate after the ramp door was closed, but well before the plane departed, and was not permitted to get on the flight. To my mind, the courtesy that we received was not necessarily mandated by the airline personnel's job description. Rather, it was a reflection of the caring of individuals who effectively communicated with each other.

I believe that apt comparisons can be made between beleaguered airline personnel and health care providers. In both occupations, work is complicated by multiple stressors. In medicine, not only are diagnoses frequently elusive, but patients and families can appear unreasonable and demanding. Tension can abound. In the face of this maelstrom, we deliver the best care when we are calm and courteous to our professional colleagues, as well as our patients and their families. Working as a team, we can most expeditiously design and implement a plan of care. It seems to me that the airline personnel in Denver demonstrated the type of collegiality I am advocating. One individual alone could not have succeeded in holding our plane until we arrived. The concerted effort of a team of individuals, who cared sufficiently for our plight, assured that their system responded to our needs. Similarly, in medicine, common courtesies among colleagues can make a difference in the care that is afforded patients. Of course the hardest times to exhibit empathy are when we are most stressed. But those occasions are precisely when courtesy and common decency count the most!

What Were We Thinking?

To regret is to be human, I suppose. I know of no one who cannot name some things that should have been done differently. Or perhaps not at all. We yearn for foresight of the future, but are fated to deal with life's realities as they unfold.

When my family and I moved to the country some twenty-five years ago, there were some things we wanted to change immediately. We had legions of sturdy burr oak, but not so many trees as we thought desirable. There were several places where we longed for "instant trees." Absent that, we wanted a species that would be fast growing and abundant. Our friends, the Bechtolds, had some giant trees that they assured us were fast growing. In fairness, they also pointed out that these trees spread prolifically by their shallow roots. In our eagerness to expand our woods, we did not closely attend to this latter disclaimer. We eagerly dug up multiple offshoots of the main trees that had "suckered up" in an adjoining field, planted them, and impatiently awaited results. In several brief years, the trees began to assume some stature. Now, years later, some of them tower forty feet or more.

Unfortunately, the predictable legacy of these trees has accompanied them. Beneath these great trees, and spreading out in all directions, new suckers are sprouting up. They are incredibly resilient as they invade a lawn. As quickly as they are mowed over, they seem to reappear. They are indomitable. As I walk through our west lawn, they are everywhere, a cancer and a plague combined. More than once, I have asked myself in recent years "What were we thinking?" When my wife and I first started planting these "Bechtold trees," we knew how they spread. However that seemed to be a secondary consideration to getting hardy trees quickly established.

I suppose one can draw an apt parallel between our having planted these trees and a person's cavalier assumption of various health risks. One does not have to look far to extend the analogy—smoking, obesity, excessive alcohol consumption, and the lack of exercise all fit the bill. Clearly there are attractions to such risky behavior, just as the "Bechtold trees" offered the appeal of availability, ease of transplanting and prospects for rapid growth. And like our battle with the ever emerging "suckers" of the original trees, physicians can find themselves waging battle after battle against the relentless onslaught of diseases caused by life-style choices.

Today our progenitor trees are magnificent. They have a sleek gray bark and green and silver leaves that shimmer in the breeze and sunlight. They continue to grow taller, far surpassing the plodding oak trees that preceded them. And thus far, we have managed to curtail the relentless spread of their offspring. That means very frequent mowing of the lawn, as well as hand pruning to remove hardy specimens from among rocks and other shrubs. This struggle can be costly in terms of time and consequence. On more than one occasion, we have discovered ourselves amid poison ivy as we worked to sever intrepid suckers.

If I could roll the clock back, we would never have planted any "Bechtold trees." But perhaps their lesson is saving me from some future folly. And, presumably, some of the afflictions that our patients endure can serve to prevent them from adopting behaviors that could cause more serious calamity. But such reflections seem mostly like after-the-fact rationalization. I still wish I'd never advocated planting those darn Bechtold trees, or ever smoked a pipe in my callow youth, for that matter.

Scythe Stories

In the clinical realm, most of what we do is premised on factual analysis and scientific data. But of course there are instances when a leap of intuition provides the solution to a problem. Presumably this is true in many realms of human endeavor.

For some time my wife had been advocating a handrail for the three steps that lead up to our front porch. Neither of us could envision a particularly creative way to accomplish this. Mary, in particular, became resigned to the fact that the handrail was a necessary concession to safety, but would detract from the appearance of the porch.

After periodically deliberating (and procrastinating) on this project, she had the opportunity to pose the perplexity to her father, Francis, during a recent visit. Pausing for a brief consideration, he asked if we had an old scythe. After quickly inspecting it, he proclaimed a solution to the problem—namely a handrail fashioned from the scythe handle, properly called the snath. He stressed that the wood used in an implement handle is sturdy ash, and then opined that the gentle curve of the snath would be both visually appealing and functional. Fortunately for us, Francis proceeded to prove his contention. He removed the two wooden grips from the shaft of the scythe and used their hardware to attach two perpendicular poles to serve as balusters for the scythe shaft. After careful deliberation as to proper material for these balusters, he settled on the handles from two old snow shovels. Like the scythe itself, these shovel handles were weathered and appropriately sturdy.

When the scythe snath had been attached to the perpendicular uprights, Francis devised one more innovation. Dulling the scythe blade on a grinder until satisfied that it was blunt as a butter knife and not likely to inflict harm to a passerby, he reattached the blade to the snath. After flexing the blade until its tip was in contact with the lower baluster, he secured it with a screw. This curved blade now served to add further stability to the assembly.

Francis' satisfaction with this creation is intriguing to me. As a skilled carpenter and craftsman he has been engaged in woodworking projects for over sixty years. But he evidences a special pride for this scythe project. He isn't sure where the idea for it came from—indeed it is almost bewildering how quickly and emphatically he suggested the scythe as a possibility for the handrail. But, he allows that this scythe-turned-handrail stands as one of his most innovative and elegant creations.

Of course, it isn't merely the appearance of the scythe handle with its graceful undulation that intrigues. To see a scythe displayed is also to evoke images of how it becomes a potent tool in skilled hands. I recall times that I have been riveted by the sight of a lone figure standing amid green as he rhythmically lays down the cut grass in neat rows. This image evokes a nostalgia for an older time, perhaps the speckled sunlight and rural settings of French Impressionism. Sturdy self reliance seems evident in the whir and scratch of the grass being laid down. To watch the scythe in action is to sense a reverence in the operator. Rhythm and precision are demanded, as are careful preparations. In centuries past, a small anvil and hammer were carried into the field in order to "draw the blade out" to sharpness after it was used for a time. Today a whetstone can be employed in circular rhythm to restore a blade to optimal function. The attentive ritual of blade maintenance is indispensable to scythe work.

I suppose that the use of the scythe—whether employed as a venerable cutting tool or adapted artistically to some unconventional function—can serve as a metaphor for human enterprise. Creativity and talent are ubiquitous if one is fortunate enough to recognize them. Being in health care certainly does not guarantee an exclusive insight into the human condition, but it can work to hone our appreciation of the possible. To the extent that we are able to marvel at human ingenuity, to relish the nuances of motivation and focus, our personal and professional lives are enhanced.

Perspective

To be in the presence of genius is to celebrate all of human potential. Over the years, I have had an opportunity to benefit from such associations. One can, of course, encounter genius in many fields. The visual arts are an excellent example. The works of Marianne Larsen and Mary Selvig, both of Sioux Falls, come to mind. Larsen's medium is photography. She has an uncanny ability to focus upon the ordinary and render it utterly appealing and extraordinary. Selvig is a potter whose elegant artistry evokes yearning and truth. She works with clay and other naturally occurring materials to effect her creations.

Another example of genius, this time in neighboring Minnesota, is John Schellinger. He is a 28 year old master woodworker whose wooden boats are breathtaking. He conceives and lofts his boats himself rather than working from others' designs. I have watched his boats being fashioned. Everything matters in his work whether it be the curve of the keel, the elegant wine-glass shape of the stern, or the precision of the lithe ribs that support the lapstrake surface of the boat.

Recently, I was at a wooden boat show with John. A few of the boats, like John's, were of contemporary construction. Many boats, however, were fifty to seventy-five years old and clearly revered by those attending the festival. It was exhilarating to watch the clusters of people standing around John's two boats and to hear them comment on the mastery of his work. At one point, while we were standing off to the side, John wondered where his Whitehall boat would be a hundred years from now. He asked the question matter-of-factly and without a hint of hubris. He was simply quietly acknowledging the skill he possesses and the fact that there is a high likelihood that successive generations will revere and preserve his boats.

In the days that followed, I continued to ponder John's query as to the future fate of his artistry. I was struck by his prescience in even asking the question, and I vaguely entertained a parallel with medical practice. Several days after the boat show, I was engaged in quiet conversation with another physician whom I have always respected. As we talked, I found myself thinking of his work as a form of artistry not dissimilar to the creativity of Schellinger or Larsen or Selvig. Specifically, my friend and I pondered the challenges of hospital practice. He casually remarked how much he valued working with patients and families in crisis. His words seemed carefully chosen, and I urged him to elaborate. In particular, he stressed that he feels himself called to work with people in the most trying circumstances. He further clarified that even those patients and families who are particularly demanding and unhappy can prove gratifying.

It seems to me that most physicians rue such conflict. Difficult patients can be particularly troubling. I have known times when I thought it fortunate to have looked into a hospital room and discovered that the hovering family had just left for lunch. Virtually all family encounters prolong a hospital visit, and there are times when family interaction can heighten physician anxiety and frustration.

Recently, on a weekend, I had an initial visit with an elderly man suffering from a bad stroke. Forty-eight hours after the onset of his symptoms he still had a severe speech disturbance and paralysis. Clearly, he was not destined to do well. I sat down with twelve family members and went through his tests and why I felt his stroke was so severe. The family posed question after question. At the conclusion of our meeting, as they stood to leave, one daughter asked her brother if he had any more questions. "No," he said "not really. All the answers that we heard today are the same ones our doctors told us yesterday."

This type of encounter is not unusual or profound. It exemplifies, however, the challenges in dealing with the patients and their families. They cling to our explanations and the nuances implied. Certainly some patients and families, although concerned, readily accept our diagnosis and prognostications. Others seem to instinctively adopt an adversarial tone and to question medical recommendations at every turn.

41

What impresses me about my physician friend is that he seems truly at ease dealing with the range of human emotions. He readily acknowledges that the care of patients and families is exceedingly difficult. But he seems able to accept and even embrace this as an integral part of his profession. Since he has practiced for many years, his reflections are not glibly made. Rather, he seems to be energized and inspired by the social complexities he encounters. His attitude reminds me of passages from William Carlos Williams' *Doctor Stories*. In discussing a home visit in which he encounters a spouse and patient, Williams almost bubbles over with enthusiasm. When first asked if he would make the visit he exclaims, "Would I!," acknowledging his eagerness to be involved. As he enters the home, he relishes the privilege, exclaiming "what a thrill I got!"[1] Williams clearly loved his work as a physician, and I believe my friend does also. Attitude is important here. My friend readily acknowledges that he can be challenged and stressed in the course of providing hospital care. However, he seems to have carefully anticipated this eventuality and prepared for it.

From time to time, I believe most physicians need an adjustment of attitude. All too readily we can develop feelings of being overburdened. The incessant demands and frustrations that we encounter can easily take a toll on our outlook. It helps, I think, to repeatedly remind ourselves that our work is unavoidably demanding. Often we encounter people who can seem ungrateful and obstreperous. We are best able to tolerate the difficulties of our profession if we allow ourselves to be fascinated by the opportunity to enter into the intimacies of people's lives. Creativity and perseverance are also required.

It seems to me that the artistry of medicine has the same type of long term implications that were being pondered by the boat builder, Schellinger. To the extent that we are able to decisively intervene in patients' lives, we caregivers can create an enduring legacy. I actually do recall the name of my grandfather's kindly physician. His personality and healing presence had an impact on my mother and ultimately on the lives of my siblings and me. Stories of healing and caring are cherished and can be passed on either explicitly or implicitly. Thus, the repercussions of what physicians accomplish in the clinical realm today may well be felt by generations of the future. While this type of clinical artistry obviously lacks the visual permanence of a wooden boat or a sculpture, it can endure in more subtle ways.

In the face of the insistent demands of daily medical practice, a caregiver can become hardened and fatigued. Certainly it is possible to mistake clinical work as being merely a mechanism to achieve a secure livelihood. But to the extent that we caregivers see ourselves as artists—a profession challenged to traverse the difficult terrain of human emotion with sensitivity and skill—we can embrace the thrill and privilege of what we do.

References
[1] Williams WC. Ancient Gentility. In: Doctor Stories. New York: New Directions; 1932.

A Death Foretold

Over the years, I have remembered fondly certain literary works and phrases, or at least paraphrases of them. On those occasions when I have actually returned to the original source, I have discovered that my memory of the exact quotations and context is sometimes errant. When I decided to write some reflections on a dying patient, I recalled Faulkner's Nobel Prize winning book, *As I Lay Dying*.[1] I remembered the book's first scene beginning with a woman dying while a carpenter builds her casket outside the bedroom window. When I actually perused the novel again, I discovered I didn't have it precisely right. The book is written in very short chapters, and the scene I recalled as beginning the book is actually developed in three different chapters. Quotations from these chapters do, however, flow together and provide a flavor of Faulkner's writing and messages:

> "Standing in a litter of chips, he is fitting two of the boards together. Between the shadow spaces they are yellow as gold, like soft gold, bearing on their flanks in smooth undulations the marks of the adze blade: a good carpenter, Cash is. He holds the two planks on the trestle, fitted along the edges in a quarter of the finished box. He kneels and squints along the edge of them, then lowers them and takes up the adze. A good carpenter. Addie Burdren could not want for a better one, a better box to lie in.
>
> The quilt is drawn up to her chin, hot as it is, with only her two hands and face outside. She is propped up on the pillow, with her head raised so she can see out the window, and we can hear him every time he takes up the adze or the saw. If we were deaf we could almost watch her face and hear him, see him.

It's because he stays out there, right under
the window, hammering and sawing on that
goddamn box. Where she's got to see him.
Where every breath she draws in is full of his
knocking and sawing where she can see him
saying See. See what a good one I am making
for you." [1]

My thoughts of Faulkner were prompted by a woman I
knew who lay dying for over a year. I will refer to her as
Summer Olsen, a pseudonym she actually adopted for a brief
period as a young woman. Summer's health had been devastated by a series of strokes. Her speech became slow and difficult to understand. She manipulated her arms with difficulty
and had no functional use of her legs. At fifty, Summer was
suffering the ravages of her juvenile onset diabetes mellitus.
She entered a hospice program, expressing little interest in the
world around her and seemingly anxious to die. Initially, several hospice volunteers alternated visits with her. Eventually
one of them, Mary, opted to begin seeing her on a consistent,
daily basis. They became good friends. To pass the hours of
forced immobility, Mary began to read to Summer. These
readings included a mystery/adventure series by a popular
author. Summer became engrossed in these stories. She frequently talked and joked about the characters and encouraged
other family members and acquaintances to read the books.
Summer even claimed to dream about the characters and their
predicaments. After they had completed the first six books in
the series, Summer and Mary waited eagerly for the seventh
volume to be published. Mary completed reading it to her days
before Summer finally died.
    It seems to me that during this year, Mary's involvement
with Summer enabled her to move beyond simply waiting to
die like Faulkner's character. Through the vehicle of their
friendship and the series of seven books read aloud, Summer
seemed to gain a sense of renewed interest in living. While she
still railed against her neurologic impairments and forced lim-

itations, Summer also laughed frequently and very much enjoyed the companionship of sharing these stories. These activities seemed to enable Summer to continue to participate in life rather than to merely await death.

In this context, I am reminded of an emphasis championed by Dr. Arthur Olsen, a Professor of Bioethics at Augustana College and USD Medical School. Invoking the spirit of the theologian, Karl Barth, Olsen emphasizes the importance of each person living out his or her "life story." Oftentimes, that process can assume unanticipated aspects in the face of serious illness and impending death. Stories to this effect are included in the text, *The Call to Care*, that Olsen helped edit. For instance, oncology nurse Sue Halbritter vividly recounts the story of how a husband, not wanting to see his wife suffer with end-stage cancer, requested something to hasten her death. Later, however, this husband expressed feelings of gratitude that his request had not been honored and that he and his wife had the opportunity to spend her final days together. During this time, they savored their expressions of love and concern for each other, and they addressed important family issues. Of their final two weeks together the husband noted, "You know, she had a lot of work she needed to do."[2]

Simone De Beauvoir wrote a short novel entitled, *A Very Easy Death*.[3] As the work proceeds, it becomes evident that the title is meant to be ironic. In fact, the elderly French woman who is dying has a difficult and demeaning course. The events of her final days are notably different from those of Halbritter's narrative in which a dying wife and her husband are able to accomplish much of importance in the final days. Even for this couple, however, it seems inaccurate to characterize the wife's death as "easy." Unfortunately, some people are not only denied an easy death but also the ability to live out a life story in a meaningful and dignified way. Mary, the hospice volunteer, helped transform a dying experience. We caregivers are fortunate when given such an opportunity. Sometimes we can truly help a patient to complete a life story rather than to merely succumb to inevitable death. Mary clearly succeeded in this effort. By reading to Summer, and otherwise making her feel that she was of primary importance, I believe Mary enabled her to find aspects of living that could be relished even in the face of a death foretold.

The term "death with dignity" is frequently invoked to describe what we, individually and collectively, hope for. Of the gifts we offer each other, as professionals and friends, perhaps the most appreciated is our time. Being there can make all the difference. It is sufficient and enduring.

References

[1] Faulkner W. As I Lay Dying. New York: Vintage; 1930, 1957.

[2] Olsen A, Freeman JW, Auterman M, Robinson R, editors. The Call to Care. Sioux Falls: Ex Machina; 1999.

[3] De Beauvoir S. A Very Easy Death. Westminster: Pantheon Books; 1965.

Risk Taking

Recently, I heard a radio interview with a songwriter who expressed an ongoing fear that her creativity might become stifled. She recounted that while working on her last album, she had devised a tune but went for days unable to compose appropriate lyrics. She worried that the words might never come.

Presumably, many people suffer similar pangs of uncertainty. I know I have. In fact, many times after crafting some poetry I am satisfied with, I wonder where in the world I will come up with an idea for a next piece or the one after that. While creativity may become arrested, the fear of that happening exceeds the likelihood, at least in many cases. However, there certainly are a number of examples in literature in which a writer created a magnum opus and then subsequently never again exhibited similar genius. I wonder if this was the case with Harper Lee after she wrote *To Kill A Mockingbird*. Or perhaps this happened to Margaret Mitchell after writing *Gone With The Wind*.

In any event, I think that the trepidations and uncertainties of the literary artist may well parallel those of the physician. Especially when I am on call and notified of some pending calamity, I find it natural to worry in advance whether my diagnosis will be accurate and my recommended treatment efficacious. I don't mean to imply that I am riddled with insecurities. Indeed, aging and experience have added considerably to my confidence that I know what to do and what to avoid. Still, uncertainty in medicine abounds. Indeed, it is often inescapable.

The impact of this reality hit me forcefully as I stood in the emergency room at the bed of a 60-year old male two hours into a stroke. Although he could not speak because of aphasia, he and his wife listened intently as I went through the various therapeutic options and risks. As I made the recommendation for TPA, I found myself both metaphorically, and in reality, trying to peer into his future to decide if he would ultimately benefit from the treatment or would, within several hours, become a casualty of a complicating cerebral hemorrhage. Statistics aside, what he and his wife wanted to know, and I yearned to predict, is what differences in his life would result from this treatment. We all knew where we wanted to go but were uncertain of the route. And we remained uneasy through that first night and the days that followed. As often seems to happen, the patient and his wife wanted me to choose the best therapy after I had laid out options and statistics. Ultimately, I believe, both experience and a "gut feeling" guided my therapeutic decision. But even with all my resources at hand, I was still, in the end, left nervously waiting and hoping.

In some ways, the physician's creative impulses necessarily involve risk taking. While we want the safest and most effective options for patients, we sometimes lack the data to clearly establish how to proceed clinically. Of paramount importance, of course, is to try to limit adverse side effects and morbidity for our patients.

Some years ago, a friend reflected on the difference between risk taking and foolhardiness. He had been trying to explain this to his five-year old son as the child stood on the edge of a cabin loft and contemplated jumping. My friend, who himself has taken many calculated risks in life, tried to patiently explain to his son that while one may embark on endeavors that have some inherent risk, it is most prudent to avoid an action that is dangerously foolhardy. After my friend finished this discussion, he was feeling satisfied that he had imparted an important moral lesson to his son. Then, to his amazement, his son jumped. Fortunately, no permanent injury occurred, but my friend was mightily chagrined. This father had taken a risk that his son would adopt a parent's point of view but the child listened to his own impulses.

Similarly, physicians routinely encounter the risk of being misunderstood or unfairly blamed. A fellow physician recounted to me an event that occurred during his residency. A patient was dying, and the resident joined family members as the patient literally took her last breaths. When the cardiac monitor became flat, my friend reached up and turned it off. The family was appalled, thinking that he had "turned off life supports." And so it goes.

If we take our work seriously, we will always have some sense of apprehension about outcomes. We walk through risk-laden territory. Hopefully, we know enough and care enough to get by.

The "Think System"

At some point in the past, I began to champion the "think system." I suspect I became enamored with the concept through Meredith Wilson's *The Music Man*. In that story, the protagonist, Professor Harold Hill, urges the children of River City, Iowa, to make do without the musical instruments he'd promised but then failed to produce. He exhorts them to learn to play using the "think system." In the spirit of Hill's rhetoric, I have jokingly credited the "think system" as a method for resolving various quandaries.

When I was in medical school, I recall one classmate who, during the entirety of the first two years of lectures, sat quietly with his arms folded looking at the speaker. No one ever saw him take a single note. His serenity was in striking contrast to the rest of his classmates who were frantically trying to write down all of the salient details of each lecture. Then and now, I have a notion that this singular student had it right. He understood the "think system." He focused his attention and listened rather than being distracted by other lecture-room mechanics. His method was particularly notable because he consistently did very well on the tests.

When my son was in grade school and high school, he too found note-taking to be very tedious. From a young age, I recommended that he adopt the "think system" for the classroom. While I myself never really dared to eschew note taking, my son mastered the method. To this day he seems comfortable in listening and concentrating on a speaker rather than being caught up in an effort at futile transcription.

Of course the "think system" can be used in other settings as well. It can be applied to problem solving in general. On occasion, the method has helped me deduce a solution for something mechanical, although the odds are generally against me in such endeavors. Also, the method can be helpful in the realm of patient care. Invariably, successful use of the "think system" in the clinical world demands that we listen carefully to the patient narrative. Acquiring contextual data is a critical aspect of fashioning a solution. Happily, there are times when thoughtful listening and analysis permit a unifying explanation for a myriad of complex symptoms. Effective treatment may then proceed.

Unfortunately, the "think system" alone is sometimes not sufficient. In such instances, practical wisdom may be required. This can certainly be true in patient care, as well as in other aspects of our daily lives.

This spring, I had a land problem develop, and I attempted to resolve it with the "think system." We have a bridge that traverses a shallow ravine. It is constructed of large timbers recycled from an old railway trestle. These hefty timbers are about 24 feet long. They are very hard to move individually, and before this spring, the bridge (consisting of three timbers and a heavy oak decking) seemed immobile. However, during a torrential rain, the gully filled and the bridge floated up, becoming unseated from its stone foundation. Using the "think system," I tried mightily to envision how to move it back into place. I considered trying to jack it up but there was no place to obtain a purchase with my jack. I also naïvely thought I might be able to pull the bridge with my tractor in order to get it seated properly again. It didn't budge. Finally, I admitted the need for expert consultation. The "think system" needed to be supplemented. It took my father-in-law, Francis, several minutes of thoughtful consideration before he provided a solution. He reminded me, as he has in the past, of the revered triad of mechanical advantage: the lever, the fulcrum, and the inclined plane. For my problem, he felt the lever and fulcrum would prove sufficient. He explained how I could use them to lift the end of each beam in order to permit cleaning underneath and repositioning back onto the foundation. With this insight, the task was expeditiously accomplished, and the bridge again became functional.

On reflection, one can see parallels between my limitations of knowledge in terms of safely and effectively lifting a bridge and the personal limitations clinicians may feel when confronting a problem beyond their expertise. I believe that it is important to remind ourselves that we need fellow practitioners. Both informal "curb side" discussions, as well as formal consultations with other physicians can prove very helpful for patient care. The Latin root of the word doctor is "docere" meaning "to teach." As a profession, we should understand our mandate to be teachers not only to our patients, but also to our colleagues.

There are times in medicine when the "think system" is best done jointly. By carefully reflecting together on a difficult clinical problem and by pooling our wisdom and expertise, patient care can be benefited. Our work is difficult and challenging. As a profession, we should embrace those strategies that enhance our effectiveness.

Prairie Perspective

A friend recommended Kevin Bradt's book *Story as a Way of Knowing*.[1] The suggestion was a good one. Bradt understands that some realities of human existence are better characterized by story than by science. Story permits mystery and intrigue and can reflect the nuances of complicated human interaction. Story can give meaning to repressed fears and noble aspirations. It can capture the modulations of mood and intent. Story recognizes that much that is important in our lives is inevitably in flux.

While reflecting on the complexity of human enterprise and the associated role of story, it occurs to me that some possible parallels exist between our human lives and the Dakota prairie. Of course, momentous changes take place as one season yields to another. And even in a given season much variability and unpredictability are evident. Some years the tall grasses of the prairie—big bluestem, switch grass, indiangrass—are lavishly present at every turn. In other years, these grasses seem frustratingly sparse. The same is true for the prairie wildflowers. Some early springs witness the pasque flower and trillium in stunning abundance. Other years they seem to only grudgingly pop up for an occasional appearance. Like the spectrum of human personalities, the very names of prairie wild flowers reflect the understated diversity that reigns. In succession and together, species like yarrow, penstemon, fleabane, and coneflowers appear. And like human personalities, these varied flowers are able to stand alone as cherished individuals, or flourish in colorful concert with each other.

It is, of course, human nature to want the prairie to remain predictably resplendent. It would be gratifying if each summer's grasses and flowers rivaled the previous year's brilliant display. However, sequential seasons teach us that such desired predictability is not nature's way. Still, we humans yearn for our lives to be "just right." We hope for healthy longevity and success for our children and financial security. But like the prairie vegetation, our lives generally resist being harnessed into predictable patterns. Tragedy and disappointment insist upon periodic appearances.

Few things are as tantalizing as a welcome surprise. In patients' lives, I sometimes glimpse elements of heroism and kindness that surpass all expectation. Similarly, in the context of each season, nature may offer the unexpected. Last spring, while walking along a high bluff, I realized that the tops of the trees growing from the valley below were at my eye level and laden with blossoms. Of course, I had admired the towering basswoods before and probably even acknowledged their summer scent. However, the unanticipated discovery of the basswoods' fragrant blossoms at arms length before me, nurtured my gratitude for the unexpected and the partially hidden. But nothing remains perfect. After a week or so, the basswood blossoms began to fade. And all too quickly, the most remarkable moments of people's lives dissolve into the background of periodic frustration and disappointment. Again, the story of the prairie can be seen to parallel the stories of our lives.

In his book, Bradt emphasized that the context of an event or personal encounter invariably shapes reality. Or, to put it another way, reality becomes the result of interaction, whether intended or not. The critical data of life are not mere phenomena of existing but are the challenges inherent in interacting. In support of this premise, Bradt alludes to the "Heisenberg principle," noting that the very act of studying subatomic particles alters them. Similarly, in medicine, we see the effects of mutual encounter all the time. As a result of doctor-patient interaction, lives change, becoming more than the individual persons who existed prior to an illness.

We should nourish narrative and story in medicine, recognizing that there is much that is opaque and non-linear and hard to predict. Patients' lives are decisively altered by disease, as well as by encounters with caregivers. As physicians, we must view our power to influence with reverence and humility. Like next year's coneflowers, we have only a vague idea of how we are destined to appear or how adroitly we will function. The particulars that will ensue from our future patient encounters remain to be revealed.

References

[1] Bradt KM. Story as a Way of Knowing. Lanham: Sheed and Ward; 1997.

First Friday

For some years, a group of us have assembled on the first Friday of each month to discuss ethical and value issues that impact on health care. The fact that the meetings are at 7 a.m. and are well attended is something of a conundrum. Recently my father-in-law, Francis, was visiting from out of town and on short notice decided to attend one of our sessions. As usual, the composition of the group was diverse. It included physicians from various specialties, as well as representatives from nursing, pastoral care, counseling, and administration. On this particular morning, we talked about end-of-life issues. We discussed a narrative account of a medical student witnessing an elderly patient choosing to die. The group discussion was animated and insightful.

Later that morning, Francis was eager to talk more about the First Friday gathering. He expressed surprise that such a large and varied group of health care professionals cared enough about ethical and cultural issues to convene for an hour away from otherwise pressing schedules. He seemed genuinely impressed by this look behind the scenes.

The narrative we discussed is entitled, "Five Miles from Tomorrow." It appeared in the "Piece of My Mind" section of *JAMA* on October 18, 2000. It recounts a medical student's perspective of an elderly man in a remote arctic village who decides his usefulness to the community is at an end and that it is time for him to die. Like many narratives and our real life experiences, this account points out the complexities of interpersonal interactions and the religious and psychosocial forces that influence patients (and caregivers) in the decisions that they make.

Truth can come from unexpected quarters. As the group discussion proceeded, there certainly was a consensus that patients should have the right to participate in health care decisions impacting their lives. My medical student, who had been quietly observing, volunteered a personal anecdote. A year earlier, her father had died of an acute leukemia. Near the end

57

of his life, he had very firmly wanted continued aggressive therapy including full CPR. His physicians apparently felt strongly that no-CPR status would be better and were perceived by the family as actively lobbying to convince him of this. At one point, the doctors actually solicited his daughter, the medical student, to try to convince her father of this perspective. In the end, the student felt that although her father would not have survived long term in any event, his expressed wishes were thwarted. This personal anecdote was particularly compelling when considered in juxtaposition with the *JAMA* essay.

In offering his reflections about our Friday session, Francis seemed fascinated by the complexity and struggle that can accompany clinical decision making. He opined that it would reassure patients and families to know that caregivers devote time looking at the whole person rather than just performing the mechanics of patient care.

On that Friday morning, I do think our group was talking about the art of caregiving. Whatever we call the effort, health care providers clearly need to focus on specific patient narratives with attention to the individual subtleties that attend each person's life. We can do this in formal team sessions like our First Friday group, or in "curb side consultations" with our colleagues. The bottom line is that thoughtful deliberation is an important aspect of what we all do. It is gratifying to learn that a lay person, like Francis, feels privileged to have a glimpse of the activities that we often take for granted. The social activist, Dorothy Day, quoting a mentor who had a great impact on her life, referred to the fact that some things just "wanted doing."[1] The implication of this phrase is that in life there is a moral imperative to be of use. I believe that in medicine, our attention to the psychosocial and ethical concerns affecting our patients' lives is something that clearly wants doing. What's needed for this effort is the proper angle of vision. As a carpenter, Francis has worked with angles all his life. His sense of perspective tells him that the First Friday group was getting it right.

References

[1] Coles R. Lives of Moral Leadership. New York: Random House; 2000.

The Changing Message

Many people are familiar with the old parlor game of whispering a secret to the person at one's side and then having the softly spoken message in turn spread around a room to others. Invariably, the last person hears a considerably jumbled and sometimes grossly misconstrued version of the original statement.

Even skilled translators invariably personalize their material and necessarily render it changed from the original. Along this line, I recently compared different translations of *The Odyssey* by Homer. As demonstrated in the versions that follow, four different translators each left their unique mark as they crafted their version of Homer's opening lines.

"Sing to me of the man, Muse, the man of twists and turns driven time and again off course, once he had plundered the hallowed heights of Troy."[1]

* * * * *

"This is the story of a man, one who was never at a loss. He had traveled far in the world, after the sack of Troy, the virgin fortress . . ."[2]

* * * * *

"Sing to me, Muse, and through me tell the story of that man skilled in all ways of contending, the wanderer, harried for years on end, after he plundered the stronghold on the proud height of Troy."[3]

* * * * *

"Tell me, oh Muse, of that ingenious hero who traveled far and wide after he had sacked the famous town of Troy."[4]

Presumably, all four of these translators were very adept at rendering Homer's original Greek into English. Nonetheless, the variability in these translations demonstrates how easily we personalize data that comes under our purview. Certainly this can also be the circumstance as the physician scrutinizes a patient's clinical narrative.

As a medicine resident at General Hospital in Kansas City, Missouri, I was intrigued to learn that what a patient verbally reported did not necessarily quickly lead to the proper diagnosis. It was common in the inner city for individuals to complain about "the miseries" and "falling out spells." What these terms meant to patients seemed to vary considerably from one individual to the next. "The miseries" could refer to depression, indigestion, or bad arthritis. And "falling out spells" could pertain to a seizure, cardiac dysrhythmia, postural hypotension, or vasovagal syncope. My job, then, as it is now, was to fashion a patient's literal complaints into data pertinent to the clinical situation. There are many times when people do not precisely say what they mean. Clarification is needed to understand the subtext and the implications of literal statements.

On a popular album, entertainer Jimmy Buffett offers lyrics that capture well the sense of malleable narrative. He sings: "It's a semi-true story/Believe it or not/I made up a few things/And there's some I forgot./ But the life and the tellin'/Are both real to me . . . ."[5] In particular, Buffett's assertion that "the life and the tellin' are both real" speaks to the difficulty of discerning absolute truth. This can be evident in the clinical world, or in the realm of translators trying to dutifully convey the essence of an epic like *The Odyssey*.

As the physician enters into a patient's life and begins to grasp the dimensions of a clinical problem, the physician clearly becomes an integral part of the narrative. Some of the patient's truth becomes the caregiver's and visa versa. Repeated attempts to understand may be required. Often, we learn by successive approximations.

The poet Tennyson, in the spirit of *The Odyssey*, has Ulysses observe, "I am a part of all that I have met . . ." [6] An awesome challenge of medicine, it seems to me, is that we physicians, too, become a part of everyone with whom we interact. We are taken into patients' lives and significances, for better or worse. I suppose that this is why it is such a tragedy when we fail patients, either in fact or from the vantage of their perspective. Who we are and what we do has great significance. Patients permit us to enter secret, cherished realms and to leave our imprint there. We truly become a part of all whom we care for. Our journey, like that of the ancient Ulysses, necessarily includes some personal risk and a willingness to delve into the unknown. Despite the perils of being misunderstood or misinterpreted, we are given ever unfolding opportunities to make a difference in peoples' lives. Over and over again, we must strive to rise to the occasion.

References
[1] Fagles R, translator. The Odyssey by Homer. New York: Viking/Penguin; 1996.
[2] Rouse WHD, translator. The Odyssey by Homer. New York: New American Library; 1937.
[3] Fitzgerald R, translator. The Odyssey by Homer. New York: Vintage Classics; 1961.
[4] Butler S, translator. The Odyssey by Homer. London: Encyclopedia Britannica; 1952.
[5] Buffett J. Semi-True Story. In: Beach House on the Moon. New York: Warner Brothers; 1999.
[6] Tennyson A. Ulysses. In: Arp T, editor. Perrine's Sound and Sense. New York: Harcourt Brace: 1997.

Seeing Red

How it started is unclear. We were probably sitting around the table drinking coffee and talking about life. Perhaps one of us glanced at our Marianne Larsen photograph of the old Okaton Elevator. We might have commented on how the elevator's hardy red color endured even as the stately, wooden structure crumbled with age and neglect. At some point, I'm sure, my father-in-law, Francis, began to talk about barn-red paint. He knew the ingredients and had even mixed up a test batch in the past. All one needs is iron oxide, hydrated lime, linseed oil, and skim milk. This was the old way, he recalled, of painting barns and elevators before commercial paint was readily available and affordable.

When he came on his next visit from Minnesota, Francis pulled an old barn board from the trunk of his car. There were four neat stripes of red and brown coloration on the board—a record from a time years ago he had experimented with barn paint, seeking the right color. He also produced two quart jars of ingredients — iron oxide and hydrated lime. Now, he and I decided, the game was truly afoot. All we needed to do was find something to paint.

Mary, my wife, vetoed painting any of our existing structures barn-red, even though she professed to appreciate the color. Francis and I determined we would need to build something in order to try out the paint. I suggested a shed to cover our rows of firewood, and Francis began sketching possibilities. At one point, he and I favored an L-shaped pavilion to keep the firewood dry. It would have been splendid. But then discussion turned to a structure for the sixteen-foot Whitehall rowboat my brother-in-law had crafted for us. Gradually, this structure evolved into a boat house to be situated on the hill above our small pond. When all agreed that a red boat house was just the right thing, considerable debate commenced about the building's size and shape. Curious friends and family proffered suggestions. In the end, we adopted Francis' suggestion of a saltbox design for the building.

The painting process proved more arduous than anticipated. The thick syrupy mixture had to be repeatedly stirred and was difficult to apply. A second coat was needed, but a uniform color could not be achieved. There are various gradations of color around our building. The west side is more brilliant than the south, which sometimes has a reddish-grey tint in the sunlight. Overall, the paint has a somewhat faded and aged appearance, appropriate to a boat house.

Now, when I see red, I see mutual plans and dreams, family collaboration, and an acceptance that many of our human endeavors are not perfect. Of course, the term "seeing red" can mean different things to different people. For some, it reflects a rise to anger. For others, it connotes a certain gullibility, as in seeing the world through "rose colored glasses." Sometimes, the color red can herald gaudiness or chic. I know of one medical journal editor who probably envisions the possibility of expanding her funky footwear collection whenever she sees red.

As the Christmas holiday approaches, red can be perceived as a color that traditionally attends our celebrations of reverence and joy. This season can be a time of greeting each other with open arms and holding hands as we move forward together. It can be a time of rejoicing in the God of Abraham whose lineage has nourished the great world religions of Christianity, Judaism, and Islam. It can be a time of trying to rise above the rancor and hatred that can threaten us all.

For me, the celebration of Christmas serves to forcefully emphasize the power and potential of our lives. It is also a time to recognize our inevitable shortcomings as people of faith. We understand that adaptations and compromise will be necessary along our way. Like barn-red paint, with its beauty and imperfections, human application of religious beliefs can vary, as can our success in meeting our commitments. Hopefully, the celebration of Christmas and religious holidays of all faith traditions will help us effectively focus our noble intentions. We should cherish the promise of the possible.

Sugi's Head

Kazuaki Sugi's heads are large. The one on our porch has a diameter of 64" or so. Sugi fashioned it out of clay and fired it in the wood-fueled kiln at St. John's University a number of years ago. It is glazed in earthen tones that wax and wane depending on the ambient light. Mostly copper streaks amid shades of black seem to dominate. The ears are perfectly proportioned and lend a gentleness to the figure.

But it's the face I find most riveting as I have pondered the sculpture. The visage has intense expression, but virtually no identifiable features. There are studied indentations in the clay, but no defined nose, eyes, or mouth. It doesn't need them. The figure seems to know much more than it is willing to reveal. At dusk, undulations in the clay become solemn eyes pulling me inward to unspoken mysteries. By daylight, its expression suggests inscrutable reserve.

As I reflect on Sugi's sculpture, I find myself pondering the connections between the world of art and the intimacies of people's lives. I recall a 1998 visit to the Van Gogh exhibition at the National Gallery of Art in Washington, D.C. Even the long wait in line to see Van Gogh's paintings was engrossing. While our party, and many others, had reserved tickets weeks in advance, we still endured taxing delays before reaching the paintings. But the longest queues formed for "same-day" passes, and I was puzzled to observe that many gray, disheveled men were patiently standing in this latter line. Their blank expressions were, in retrospect, eerily like Sugi's sculpture. At first I thought that these seemingly disconsolate individuals were merely responding to the universal appeal of viewing fine art. Only later did I realize that they were waiting to pick up free tickets in order to sell them to other people who were affluent enough to disdain standing in line themselves.

Thus, the very milieu of an art exhibition can inform about human endeavor. But it is, of course, the artist and the created work itself that more predictably yield insights. In Van Gogh's life, we can readily envision how personal struggle and art can be hauntingly interwoven. While confined to his room in an asylum, Van Gogh continued to paint, creating such works as the serene "Wheatfield with a Reaper." Even while being ravaged by depression, his artistic talent was able to prevail as he gazed through the barred window of the institution.

A regional artist, Sheila Agee, has used her art to more explicitly study the paradox and tragedy that can fill our lives. Her 1998 exhibition entitled "Heaven on Earth, Hell on Earth" dramatically contrasted the serenity of nature with the turmoil, suffering, and evil that plagues the lives of many people. The Agee exhibition was effectively analyzed in Dr. Ann Pederson's book, *Where in the World is God?*[1] Pederson wrote of the "dissonant juxtaposition" portrayed in the exhibition and expressed feelings of "dynamism, instability and ambiguity" while pondering Agee's visual representations of complex and often fractured lives.

While Agee's exhibition was almost brutally explicit, certainly much of art and human endeavor is shrouded in obscurity. Again, I envision Sugi's head and think of the times that I have peered at patients trying to discern what hidden mysteries were causing their symptoms. Sometimes I have yearned to know just the simple truth of whether the patient's symptoms were purely organic or somatoform in nature. Despite my anxiety and focused intent, there have been instances when my riveted gaze has been met with the same type of veiled reserve that Sugi's sculpture suggests. It is almost as if my intense queries are reflected back to me without penetrating the subject.

On first glance, Sugi's sculpture may seem too abstract to bear witness to human experience. However, an attentive focus on the serene clay visage seems to yield hidden meanings proportionate to the observer's efforts. Perhaps such attention to Sugi's work serves as a paradigm for the effort needed to optimally appreciate another person's burden. And as a companion issue, it is logical to move to additional queries: How do we see ourselves? Who are we? Where are we headed?

The pathos evident in art and in life offers us possibilities to expand our perspectives. The success of our endeavors often depends on the effort we expend to define truth in the shadows of otherwise ordinary sunlight.

References

[1] Pederson A. Where in the World is God? St Louis: Chalice Press; 1998.

Wishful Thinking

From time to time I see patients who request a "total body scan." These persons seem to have the hope that a CAT scan or MRI can literally image them from head to toe and assure them that no problem exists. Frequently, a patient who requests such a radiologic inspection is among the "worried well," or at least among those who are not too sick. Such individuals seem to have the notion that if no tumor or blight is detected at a given time then they can truly be assured that they are in good health. There is great security in knowing that everything is as it should be. And, of course, there is the companion hope and expectation that a healthy, steady state will be indefinitely maintained into the distant future.

Often, when I am working on our family's land in rural Brandon, I ponder both the innocent inclination and the futility of seeking to maintain the status quo. Of course, we enthusiastically try to fashion things just as we want them. There are trails to mow, trees to prune, and Canadian thistles to thwart. But as we engage in these tasks, it is readily evident that all of our efforts are temporary remedies, at best. The Dakota prairie is not static and certainly does not maintain a single reality of perfection. Some years are better than others. This summer, with sufficient moisture, the grasses were verdant and flowers popped up everywhere. But nature always seems to be breaking down and changing. The native grasses are steadily invaded by buffalo berry and plum. And small oak trees continue to tiptoe slowly into the grasses, foretelling of a future time when the forest may substantially replace much of our grassland. The pond, once clear and pristine, now nourishes thick duckweed and cattails. With each fierce wind, invariably some mature trees succumb, losing large branches and sometimes splitting at the trunk.

While we gamely do battle with each disruption, it is with the sense that we are only briefly forestalling an inexorable metamorphosis. The land is resplendent in its beauty but never static. In a different context, the poet Ann Sexton finds herself "wondering how anything fragile survives…"[1] Meanwhile, we yearn for an agreeable stability that is not fragile. But the prairie cannot be fashioned to our notions of the ideal. Change is everywhere.

As physicians we understand that nothing is static. There is no flawless state of health unmarred by aches or anxiety or pathology too incipient to detect. Anatomic variations and debate about what the range of normal includes are issues that confound us. In a recent *JAMA* article, a thousand healthy volunteers underwent MRI scanning of the head. In 18% of them, some abnormalities were found. Many of these were minor, incidental findings. But a number of more notable abnormalities were uncovered, including asymptomatic tumors, vascular lesions, and possible multiple sclerosis.[2]

Presumably, for some of the individuals in the MRI study, the reality of discovering incidental and minor abnormalities provided little more than the thorn of uncertainty. We all know that the body is not perfect. But it certainly is nice to presume that nothing is wrong. When a defect or an enigma is pointed out, it is hard for any of us not to feel vulnerable and uneasy. Invariably a loss of innocence occurs as an individual is forced to confront the prospect of frailty and decline. Linda Pastan, in her poem "After minor surgery ," reflects on the human delusion of being invincible as she describes a time "when the body in all its fear and cunning makes promises to me it knows it cannot keep."[3]

There is a part of me that wants to share all these thoughts and more with the patient who requests a total body scan. But mainly, I just respond by stressing the expense and impracticality of scanning everything. Yet my inclination, what I almost say, is that absolute assurances and personal tranquility will always elude us. Naturally, we should try to adopt healthy life-styles and diligently respond to the warning signs of disease when they occur. But as physicians, we of course know that "all the time, some end lies waiting to happen."[4]

References

[1] Sexton A. The Abortion. In:The Complete Poems. Boston: Houghton, Mifflin Co.; 1981.

[2] Katzman GL et al. Incidental findings on brain magnetic resonance imaging from 1000 asymptomatic volunteers. JAMA. 1999 July 7 : 282:36-39.

[3] Pastan L. After minor surgery. In: Thomas Arp, editor. Perine's Sound and Sense. Boston: Harcourt Brace; 1997.

[4] Freeman J. Apocalypse. In: Starting from Here. Sioux Falls: Ex Machina; 1996.

Cloning and *The Odyssey*

As news of the first successfully cloned mammal emerged from Scotland, debate began to rage in the press, between politicians, and among concerned persons everywhere. With the birth and survival of one hapless sheep, still another barrier to human endeavor had been summarily transcended. At the time I began to learn of this marvel and to consider varying critiques of this stunning technology, I also happened to be reading a new translation of Homer's *The Odyssey*. Very quickly, connections and metaphors became apparent.

No one knows the precise age of *The Odyssey*, but it is estimated to have been written in about 700 B.C. and to describe events which may have transpired as early as 1200 B.C. In reading a new translation by Fagles, I was amazed at how engrossing the story remains.[1] All manner of human heroism and kindness arc mixed up with deceits and treacheries. Evil abounds. Homer's survivors of the Trojan War and their contemporaries struggled to achieve measures of justice and happiness. In Homer's day, the whims of fate were often attributed to the gods. Indeed, Homer has Zeus comment on this as follows:

> "Ah how shameless the way these mortals
> blame the gods. From us alone, they say come
> all their miseries, yes, but they themselves,
> with their own reckless ways, compound their
> pains beyond their proper share."[2]

Still today, humankind struggles to reckon with the forces we only partially control in an imperfect world. Many times we are tempted to throw up our collective hands at the futility of trying to control evil and happenstance.

In some ways, the technology for cloning (specifically the prospect of cloning human beings) may be seen as a fearsome threat to the very fabric of our human existence. Indeed, by analogy, the risks posed by the unbridled use of such technol-

71

ogy may be seen as comparable to the various terrors that confronted Ulysses as he strove to return to the comfort and security of his homeland. For instance, the allure of the Sirens had dreadful pitfalls for sailors who heard their beautiful songs and were lured into captivity. Similarly, our society may be confronting the perilous allure of technological sirens, and we may be morally too naïve to deal with the implications (*i.e.*, of genetic manipulation). However, I think it is unlikely that either government regulations or moral mandates will succeed for long in restricting such types of scientific research. It is almost as if there is an inexorable mandate to attain whatever can be scientifically envisioned. It reminds me somewhat of the circumstances of 1974 when some scientists called for a moratorium on the study of recombinant DNA because they feared that society was not ready for such knowledge. This moratorium was short-lived. My guess is that, similarly, there will be scientists who will forge ahead with research in cloning mammals even if it must be done clandestinely.

If this is the case, society desperately requires new heroes to guide us through this technologic morass. While Ulysses was the epitome of a great hero in an ancient era, our heroes of today and tomorrow will need to be cast in a much different mold. As human endeavor continues to force increasingly difficult ethical dilemmas, it is my belief that our greatest heroes of the future will be individuals who have the wisdom and ethical vision to articulate moral responses to these ethical quandaries and who can help shape societal consensus. One could argue that this type of leader must somehow rise above the current political, cultural, and religious divisiveness that seems to characterize today's society. While such a person may not be engaged in the physical dangers of warfare and exploration like Ulysses, a leader of this ilk may need the resourcefulness of that ancient hero to make sense of incredibly complex ethical issues. An older translation of *The Odyssey* by Rouse begins by describing Ulysses as, "One who was never at a loss."[3] Our visionaries of the future must possess that type of resourcefulness. In the face of seemingly

72

impossible conflicts, society will need to make fearsome compromises and choices as we progress along the course of human potential.

To reiterate, it would certainly be safest if the cloning of mammals was deferred for an indefinite period of time to enable society to catch its breath and carefully analyze whether such research should proceed. I suspect we may have a brief moratorium, but certainly not a permanent cessation, of such genetic exploration. As physicians, I believe we want to remain actively informed about such scientific and ethical issues and to firmly lend our voices to the societal discussions that will ensue. Perhaps we can help educate the women and men who will become the moral heroes of tomorrow.

References

[1] Fagles R, translator. The Odyssey by Homer. New York: Viking/Penguin; 1996.
[2] Ibid.
[3] Rouse WHD, translator. The Odyssey by Homer. New York: The New American Library; 1937.

Calamity and Caring

Recently, while musing about everything and nothing juxtaposed, I recalled the time I rolled a tractor. Now that twenty years or so have passed since the episode, I don't think of it nearly as often as I previously did. However, I still do marvel that I escaped unscathed. I was going across a relatively steep slope (a procedure that I knew even then was ill-advised) when the old offset International tractor became stuck. The wheels began to spin futilely as I attempted to either back up or go forward. In addition, the offset weight of the engine began to pull the tractor over. Somehow, that being a more agile time of my life, I managed to leap off the uphill side of the tractor. As I was airborne, one of the large rear wheels brushed against me. The tractor rolled multiple times into the gully below. There seems little doubt that if I had stayed with the machine (absent a roll bar, of course) I would have been very seriously injured or killed. Now, I find myself trying to imagine how life would be if I had crushed my spine and become a quadriplegic, or perhaps sustained a traumatic brain injury of some sort.

Aside from reminding me to feel very fortunate, this vivid memory also serves to evoke images of many patients over the years who have not had the good fortune to escape devastating injury or illness. While we often hear it said that "we should be thankful for our good health," it certainly is easy to take health for granted.

One person, who in the latter part of his life did not minimize his good fortune, was Raymond Carver. Carver was a very well-known poet and short story writer. He also had such devastating health complications due to alcoholism that it was anticipated by his physicians that he would die imminently from liver disease. However, Carver managed to stop drinking and then lived another ten years before developing a lung cancer with brain metastases. He wrote a poem in the last months of his life called, "Gravy." In it he says "Don't weep for me...I'm a lucky man. I've had ten years longer than I or anyone expected. Pure gravy. And don't forget it."[1]

In his final decade, he remarried and was very productive as a writer. He remained deeply appreciative for the gift of having thwarted what seemed to be a certain demise from alcoholism.

In a somewhat similar vein, I am reminded of a quotation from Gaylin *et al.* They note, in commenting upon the inevitable transitions of life, "If we are fortunate enough to achieve power and relative independence along the way it is a transient and passing glory, and it would be well to keep clearly in mind our inevitable decline as we contract and deal with the helpless and dependent who come within our influence."[2]

I'm intrigued by how easy it is for caregivers to become immune, or at least distanced, from the personal tragedies encountered in regular practice. Sometimes physicians act as if patients are totally responsible for the calamities that befall them, or if not responsible, then perhaps just weak links in the evolutionary chain of otherwise self-sufficient and productive human beings. Of course, Gaylin's quote serves to remind us that we all move variably through phases of dependence, independence, and back again. And Carver urges us to cherish and nurture the time we are allotted. But it is hard to always savor the good in our lives, and it is even harder to truly see ourselves as being essentially on the same continuum as our patients. John Donne wrote: "No man is an island, entire of itself; every man is a piece of the continent, a part of the main: if a clod be washed away by the sea, Europe is the less...; any man's death diminishes me, because I am involved in mankind; and therefore never send to know for whom the bell tolls; it tolls for thee."[3] Such a concept of shared destiny certainly does not inform all basic human interaction. And in the case of the caregiver, a shared human destiny does not necessarily ensure that patients are always treated with empathy and understanding for their plight.

Such reflections presuppose that all of us, at least at difficult times in our clinical practice, treat patients more casually than they deserve. When we are rushed or preoccupied or angry, it is easy to forget that our encounter with a patient may be the most significant event in that person's day. Focused awareness does not always dominate the caregiver's consciousness. Few of us can live and practice while constantly demonstrating the utmost compassion.

In his novel *The Idiot*, Fyodor Dostoevsky sheds insight upon our failures to live the lives we intend. By analogy, his story might apply to the caregiver who falls short of an earnest intention to focus resolutely on the needs of each patient. Dostoevsky tells of a prisoner who is led from his cell and sentenced to be shot. The condemned man revels in the last five minutes he has to live. He carefully portions his limited time to care for his comrades, to think, and to look about him. Later he recalls having precisely divided his remaining time and thinking: "What if I were not to die! What if I could go back to life—what eternity! And it would all be mine! I would turn every minute into an age; I would lose nothing, I would count every minute as it passed, I would not waste one."[4] But when this man is granted a reprieve from execution, he subsequently discovers that it is not possible to live with such intense appreciation of each moment. And similarly caregivers, despite the best of intentions, often fail to meet their own expectations.

And so it goes in the daily effort to get by, or to make a positive difference in people's lives. As physicians, we do what we do, some days more elegantly and compassionately than others. We realize that it is sometimes impossible for the caregiver to interact with optimal sensitivity to each patient. At times we recall that any of the illnesses we encounter in our patients could have been afflicted upon ourselves. This notion can serve simultaneously as a challenge and a cautionary tale. On that intuitive level, it does seem appropriate that the care we extend to others might anticipate our own fate.

References

[1] Carver R. Gravy. In: A New Path to the Waterfall. New York: Atlantic Monthly; 1989.

[2] Gaylin W, Glasser I, et al. Doing Good: The Limits of Benevolence. New York: Pantheon; 1978.

[3] Donne J. Devotions Upon Emergent Occasions, 1624.

[4] Dostoevsky F. The Idiot. New York: Bantam; 1958.

A Little Bit of Luck

Many diagnoses in medicine are straightforward and certain. Other times, we see persons with odd constellations of symptoms that are baffling from the onset and often remain enigmas even after extensive testing. And a most vexing patient category presents with common symptomatology as a herald of some type of rare pathology. Recently I saw two people in this latter category.

A 25 year old male presented with a severe headache of several days duration. He had a family history for migraine. After a CAT scan and spinal fluid examination were normal, treatment was started for a presumed migraine. When he did not improve a MRI of the brain was performed. This revealed a mass in the pituitary gland. It appeared that he had sustained a hemorrhage into the pituitary.

A second patient, a 23 year old woman, also had persistent headache. In her case, it began after being struck in the jaw with a softball. Her jaw had been fractured and immobilized. However her headaches persisted over several weeks. A CAT scan of the head showed subtle changes, and a subsequent MRI study of the brain confirmed extensive blood clots — so-called cerebral vein thrombosis. She was started on anticoagulation and steadily improved.

In both of these instances, young patients presented with fairly nondescript headaches. In the case of the young man, a presumption of an initial migraine headache seemed very reasonable. With the young woman, because of the trauma to her face, it seemed important to exclude bleeding to the brain. However, her presentation was not felt to be necessarily typical for cerebral vein thrombosis.

These two individuals could have experienced dire consequences if their conditions had not been diagnosed and appropriately treated. For instance, in a stressful situation, a person with a severe pituitary problem can become critically ill. In the case of cerebral vein thrombosis, one can see extensive cerebral ischemic injury, hemorrhage, or even death.

Both patients were atypical in their presentation. Pituitary hemorrhage manifesting as headache and cerebral vein thrombosis are both very unusual. Establishing an appropriate diagnosis in such patients can be particularly challenging since the prevalence of headache is so great. A majority of the population has headaches at sometime in their life.

Perhaps the best clue in both of these patients was that their headaches were new and unusual for them. Such circumstance warrants further evaluation. But even the clinical decision to obtain brain imaging did not guarantee that a diagnosis would be promptly made. In the case of the young woman with cerebral vein thrombosis, the CAT scan was initially interpreted as normal. It was only after I remained uneasy about her clinical picture that subtle CAT scan abnormalities were appreciated and a definitive MRI ordered. Similarly, in the case of the young man with pituitary tumor, an initial CAT scan was non-diagnostic. When the MRI was ordered, I was not at all sure that any additional pathology would be discovered, especially since his headache continued to act like migraine.

For both of these patients, a correct diagnosis was reached fairly quickly and appropriate treatment initiated. However, both cases prompt me to experience a sense of disquietude. The actual pathologic culprit was not initially considered in either patient. And it is unsettling to think that sometimes we caregivers end up looking brilliant by virtue of happenstance and good fortune. All of us would much prefer that our diagnoses result from exquisitely focused deductions. Yet, there do seem to be times when clinical acumen is aided by fortuitous developments.

Unfortunately, neither the severity of a headache nor its location definitively establishes a diagnosis. For instance, a patient with classic migraine could appear to be in much more severe pain than a person with a ruptured aneurysm. In addition, although migraine is classically hemicranial, it can present in a variety of locations.

Such clinical cases can serve as a cautionary tale against clinical arrogance. Mistakes are everywhere waiting to happen. Even in the case of a seasoned clinician, it sometimes takes at least some element of fortuitousness to achieve the ultimate diagnosis. Of course, none of us like to think that our clinical acumen sometimes requires serendipity and good fortune. But given the vagueness of diagnosis and the unpredictable responses to treatment, most experienced clinicians are unwilling to dismiss good fortune (or blind luck) from their clinical armamentarium.

Theater and Medicine

My wife and I went to St. Paul to attend an opera. Upon arriving in the downtown area, we discovered unexpected bustle and excitement. Serendipitously, we found ourselves in the midst of the St. Paul Winter Carnival. The citizens of St. Paul have been making the best of dreary winters with this festive celebration for well over a hundred years. Apparently, the idea for a winter celebration was initiated after a visiting *New York Times* journalist noted, in 1885, that St. Paul was the Siberia of North America and unfit for human habitation. On the weekend we visited, the temperature hovered around -5°, but that did not prevent citizens and visitors from enjoying a number of wintertime festivities. There is an aspect of ongoing theater with this celebration in that every year individuals are designated to act out roles from the legendary winter realm of Boreas. Thus a king, queen, princesses, and other personalities roam through the downtown area in costume, acting out their parts. Much of the time they congregate in Rice Park, the site of elaborate ice sculptures and carvings created each year.

The opera we attended, Verdi's *La Traviata*, was obviously theater on a more formal order. The production was presented in the Ordway Theater, just across the street from the Winter Carnival festivities in Rice Park. I was interested to learn that Verdi's work was deemed a dismal failure when initially performed in 1853. Indeed, the first audiences apparently viewed it as bleakly as the *New York Times* journalist viewed frigid St. Paul. However, when the opera was reintroduced a year later, it was much heralded and has since been an enduring favorite of audiences.

A writer of essays must be constantly on the lookout for subject matter. To this end, I pondered whether a juxtaposition of the Winter Carnival and *La Traviata* could lend itself to reflections upon medicine. My initial idea (later discarded) involved musing on how individuals can overcome the adversities of illness to lead restored (and sometimes enhanced) lives. By analogy, the citizens of St. Paul fashioned such a res-

81

urrection from the disparaging comments of a journalist and the reality of Minnesota winters. And Verdi, by dint of persistence and hope, succeeded in resurrecting *La Traviata* from a critical failure to a widely acclaimed success.

However, I became distracted from this line of reflection when I noted in the opera program that the original director of the current version of *La Traviata*, Jonathan Miller, was trained as a physician. He is described in the program notes as being "a true Renaissance man." In addition to his medical background, he is credited with being a philosopher, author, lecturer, film and theater director, and television personality.[1] A library search of Miller yielded the data that he practiced medicine briefly, but has mainly fashioned a career in television and theater. He is referenced in two interesting articles on medical practice and acting that appeared in a 1994 issue of the medical journal *Lancet*. A commentary entitled "Department of Theatrical Medicine?" makes the point that theater and medicine have long had some connection. As examples of this premise, the article notes that Chekhov and Somerset Maugham were physicians who wrote plays; Moliere and George Bernard Shaw wrote plays about doctors; and Shakespeare apparently had an intimate knowledge of medicine.[2] In the same issue, the article "Acting in Medical Practice," asserts that acting is a central feature of effective medical care. The premise is advanced that acting should be specifically taught in medical schools.[3] To substantiate this argument, the author uses the example that it is generally important for the physician to be encouraging and hopeful to patients with chronic illness. The physician needs to espouse a cheerful and positive perspective regardless of his or her frame of mind that day. The author notes that even if the physician is out of sorts because of personal factors (such as fatigue, anger, or concern about a family issue), the physician must still attempt to be responsive and attentive to the patient at hand.

To espouse acting, as such, as a part of medical education and patient care seems somewhat risky. Certainly, physicians could rightly oppose "acting" to the extent that it deceives patients, impairs patient autonomy, or misrepresents a physician's true feelings about a therapeutic issue. On the other hand, such a notable hero of modern medicine as William Osler advocated a form of theatrics in his famous Aequanimitas.[4] Osler stressed that the physician must exhibit "imperturbability." He recommends "coolness and presence of mind under all circumstances, calmness amid storm, clearness of judgement in moments of grave peril . . . and a physician who has the misfortune to be without it, who betrays indecision and worry, and who shows that he is flustered and flurried in ordinary emergencies, loses rapidly the confidence of his patients." Osler goes on to note, "the first essential is to have your nerves well in hand." Certainly this sounds like potential theatrics, especially in situations where unexpected calamity suddenly befalls a patient and urgent intervention is required. I agree with Dr. Osler that it is advisable for the physician to appear calm and collected. From experience, I suspect that some of this demeanor may well be a façade covering a turmoil of emotions brewing within the physician.

We learn medicine by a mentoring system. In addition to absorbing the scientific data of illness treatment, student physicians invariably come to emulate aspects of clinical behavior that seem particularly effective when dealing with patients. Gradually, as a result of explicit tutoring, as well as unconscious internalization of observed behaviors, the medical student and resident begin to act differently. They become more assured and confident of themselves. Most of the time, they achieve some measure of the outward equanimity espoused by Osler.

While conceding some connection between "acting" and medical practice, I am not prepared to advocate explicit instruction in "theatrical medicine." Still, I believe that self-analysis is an important attribute for individual physicians as well as the medical profession as a whole. Perhaps explicitly perceiving theatrics as an aspect of what we do may have some benefit in our ultimate understanding of ourselves. And indeed one can, without much difficulty, posit instances in medical training where acting may be explicitly beneficial. Role-playing techniques with students might enable them to refine their understanding of such difficult issues as sexual harassment, cheating, and dishonesty.

In the end, I believe the physician is invariably benefited by working to expand an understanding of the human experience. This can be in formal or informal settings. The Winter Carnival in St. Paul illustrates how theater can be used to cope with seemingly interminable winters. A splendid opera like *La Traviata* can, like other works of art, serve to champion creative potential and to portray elements of human behavior. And seeing the physician as partly engaged in theatrics can also serve to clarify the good and bad aspects of what the doctor does and how it is done. The human condition seems boundless in its range of emotional and personal responses to daily living. The physician is both a witness to, and an inevitable participant in, the everyday tumult of life and death. It seems we never know or understand enough.

References
[1] Verdi's La Traviata. In: Minnesota Opera Program. Minneapolis: Skyway; 1996.
[2] McManus C. Department of Theatrical Medicine? Lancet. 1994 Sep 17; 344: 767.
[3] Finestone HM., Counter DD. Acting in medical practice. Lancet. 1994 Sep 17; 344, 8925; 801- 802.
[4] Osler WM. Aequanimitas. 3rd Ed. Philadelphia: Blakiston; 1932.

The Bolo Tie and Minorities

It seems to me that the bolo tie is viewed as an eccentricity by many and an aberration by more critical observers. Even though there are hopeful signs that the bolo may be developing a kind of chic in some circles, this type of neck apparel remains much less in evidence than varieties of piercing and tattoos. Nonetheless, the bolo is much more of a conversation piece than most traditional silk ties.

To insert a personal perspective, let me say that I adopted the bolo quite innocently. At the orientation for my medicine residency, the Chief announced quite emphatically that male residents should always be clad in a tie. The only one I owned at the time was a small triangular bolo given to me years before by my grandfather. Since I had a slight inclination to contrariness and lacked the discretionary funds to purchase more conventional ties, I opted to wear this bolo for the next two years. The Chief occasionally looked sternly at me over his glasses but it may have been for provocations other than my apparel.

By the time I started medical practice, I had acquired several traditional silk specimens. Studied unobtrusiveness seemed best for a novice consultant. I probably did not give the fabled bolo another thought for fifteen years or so. Then, while helping sort through the various small treasures my grandparents had acquired in their combined 180 years, I came upon a turquoise bolo of Native American design that my grandfather had frequently worn. On occasion, to honor his memory, I daringly began to wear it. Then my wife bought me a second bolo and a third. Also, I again began to relish the freedom of leaving the top shirt button askew. And gradually, the search for yet another unique bolo became almost a quest of quixotic proportions. For instance, while recently traveling across the state and stopping at Al's Oasis, I spent more time studying the various snakeskin and Black Hills Gold bolo ties than I did the menu.

Frequently, a well-chosen bolo provokes comment from a stranger. Passersby on the street march over to have a closer look. Recently, a physician in the state, who had attended one of my lectures, wrote me saying, "You look a little more country than I expected. Very refreshing for a Sioux Falls doctor…" I am not certain, but I suspect he was reacting to the bolo of that day.

Once, while teaching an evening class at Augustana College, I determined to wear a different tie each night. I even kept a list for awhile so that I could remember which ties I had worn. However, I eventually became muddled in my record keeping and began to suspect that the students had more pressing things on their minds than the diversity of my tie collection.

In truth, the person adorned in a bolo usually looks a bit eccentric. And this thought leads me somewhat circuitously to the more serious subject of being in the minority, or more specifically, being Hmong. While I would hasten to stipulate that there is no close association between the Hmong in America and the intrepid bolo wearer, these two entities might be beneficially contemplated together.

Thousands of Hmong now live in this country. Many immigrated from Laos in the Vietnam War era. They continue to come and, with their large families, have begun to constitute a sizeable minority in some communities. It was estimated that Minnesota's Hmong population has probably doubled over seven years in the 1990's. In 1997 between 35,000 and 50,000 Hmong lived in the state. Minnesota is second only to California in terms of Hmong population. These numbers seem to be steadily increasing.[1]

My interest in the Hmong was piqued when a friend sent a review of the recently published book, *The Spirit Catches You and You Fall Down*.[2] This book is an elegant study of two cultures clashing in a California city—the Hmong and the medical profession of that community. The book tells the story of a young Hmong girl with intractable epilepsy. The author successfully provides the reader with perspectives from both the child's family and from the medical profession that tried earnestly, and ultimately futilely, to care for her. Huge barriers existed between these groups. The child's parents spoke very little English and poorly understood physician instructions about why medicine should be taken and how it should be used. To complicate matters, multiple different regimens were employed in an effort to stop the girl's seizures. Time and again her parents, who indisputably loved and tried to care for her, were unsuccessful in complying with physician directives about what should be done. Ultimately, after many office visits and a two-year interval that saw this child hospitalized eighteen times, she suffered severe, irreversible brain injury from a very prolonged seizure. The author of the book sensitively tries to understand what went wrong by scrutinizing the rigidity and inflexibility manifested by the physicians, the child's parents, and the extended Hmong community.

None of the Hmong in this story were reported to be wearing bolo ties. Yet, the attending physicians and residents who cared for them viewed the Hmong as essentially beyond understanding in terms of their customs and beliefs. The upshot in this California community, and potentially in other communities with large minority groups, was that organized medicine failed to be of use in an effective, consistent fashion. The misconceptions and fears of both groups inadvertently worked in concert to ensure that tragedy would ensue.

I recommend this book highly. All of us deal with minority populations. The numbers of immigrants in our cities and towns are steadily increasing. As physicians, we need to take the lead in the effort to improve understanding between cultures. And we need to ensure that our office staffs and health care institutions diligently join in our efforts.

The bolo tie can be of some small help here. It can serve as a symbol that modest eccentricity is tolerated. Indeed, the bolo might be construed as a totem to uniqueness. Whenever we see one, we can remind ourselves that being somewhat different is okay, and sometimes preferable. Besides, appreciating the rich diversity of bolo ties can be akin to relishing the uniqueness and sometimes stunning individuality of each patient we see. This is not, of course, to imply that everyone who dares to wear a bolo tie is attempting a profound social statement. I would recommend that the next time you encounter a person so attired, you should at least entertain the possibility that some profundity is waiting to be recognized.

References
[1] Bonner B. Minnesota's Population of Hmong on the Rise; Immigration Expected to Add to Other Gains. St. Paul Pioneer Press. 1997 May 5.
[2] Fadiman A. The Spirit Catches You and You Fall Down. New York: Farrar, Straus, and Giroux; 1997.

Making Change

Lately, I have been thinking about change in all its guises and about how it can come in increments or abruptly. Some weeks ago, I unilaterally effected the latter type of change in our household. I announced that we should vary the location of our artwork. Some of our art had been riveted to an assigned place since our home was built many years ago. And my wife, by her own admission, does not think much of such revisionism. Nonetheless, I was able to win a concession to try my plan based on the argument that if the rotation of artwork is an established convention for art museums, it certainly should be permissible for a household. In the end, both family and friends agreed that the artistic upheaval was a success. Since our art pieces are now in new positions, we all notice and appreciate the work much more. But when the subject comes up, my wife is quick to point out how hard the change was.

Ultimately, only some of life's inevitable changes can be construed as beneficial. It is certainly not unusual for change to leave us feeling melancholy, bereft, or angry. Instances readily come to mind. The current trend in American businesses, including health care institutions, to downsize is an excellent example. While such measures may make economic sense, they invariably result in upheavals in people's lives. Sometimes this can mean the loss of a job after working diligently for an organization for decades. At other times, individuals are moved from the security of work they have always known to totally revised job descriptions. Such wholesale change can never be accomplished without some suffering.

It occurs to me that medicine, of all endeavors, is premised on necessary change. One need look no further than the burgeoning arsenal of pharmaceuticals to know that we can only keep up in our profession by recognizing and adapting to change. However, while scientific advances can be fairly readily accepted as beneficial change, it is of course much more difficult with other types of alterations in our professional lives. The dramatic transformations effected in medicine by virtue of managed care demonstrate the challenges and frustrations inherent in fundamentally reordering human endeavor.

Of course, many of life's changes can be readily accommodated. And given the inevitability of change, it is somewhat curious how much we humans resist it. Or, to think of it in the converse, it is notable how ardently we labor to maintain the status quo. Often we are appalled by the incremental insults of aging and are capable of cursing and lamenting death, even when it follows a full and productive life. We want our children preserved and protected and often struggle as they mature and depart to exercise their independence. The poet Dylan Thomas noted that even when humans promote and encourage change, still "they grieved it on its way..."[1] As a measure of the possible deleterious effects of too much change, a scale was developed some years ago to rate a person's "life change units."[2] The presumption of this model is that persons with an excessive number of changes in a given period of time are at some emotional peril.

While thinking about change in general, I happened to be recently reminiscing with my brother about our grandfather. This kindly man adapted to many upheavals during his eighty-one years of life and served as a powerful influence for my brother and me. He wasn't perfect, and sometimes when he made a bold change it backfired. One such misstep occurred when he decided to trade in his loyal Willys jeep, a companion of many years. For some reason, he decided he wanted a new four-wheel drive vehicle. Alas, the new model lacked the character and dependability of the old jeep. My grandfather soon realized he had made a mistake. And his grandsons still rue the loss of that family jeep almost thirty years after it was traded away.

While the foregoing paragraphs have dealt with change in the sense of effecting change and adapting to it, with the title of this essay I also envisioned "making change" in another context — *i.e.* the balance or remainder after a transaction. In a fashion, we in medicine "make change" in this latter way also. That is, after a serious illness or injury has occurred, the caregiver is inevitably immersed in the effort of trying to restore meaning to what remains of a patient's life after the affliction. All of our medical efforts — surgery, medication, rehabilitation — can be construed as "making change" in this latter sense.

As physicians, we know that our profession will many times demand that we adapt to change. Clearly, that is essential to scientific advances in health care. And just as necessary is our ability to help our patients "make change" after they are afflicted with illness or injury. Simply reflecting upon the inevitability of change in these two senses does not ensure easy acceptance. Indeed, I am reminded of the line from Robert Frost's poem "Birches": "May no fate willfully misunderstand me and half grant what I wish..."[3] Too much change often threatens to overwhelm us. Yet a resource we humans collectively share is the ability to understand the meaning of change and to assimilate it into the context of our lives.

References

[1] Thomas D. Do Not Go Gentle Into That Good Night. In: Arp TR, editor. Perrine's Sound and Sense. Boston: Harcourt Brace; 1997.

[2] Rahe RH, Ryman DH, and Ward HW. Simplified Scaling for Life Change Events. Journal of Human Stress. 1980 Dec. 6(4): 22-27.

[3] Frost R. Birches. In: Robert Frost's Poems. New York: Pocket Books; 1971.

Promises Made

Quite naturally, humankind yearns for definitive cures for its physical maladies. There is probably no better paradigm for this instinct than multiple sclerosis (MS), a chronic disease that afflicts the young and middle-aged. Multiple sclerosis can cause incremental and progressive disability. Invariably, great uncertainty and apprehension exist among those afflicted. Always there is a concern about when the next flare may occur or how much disability one might suffer over the years.

One way that people cope with such uncertain prospects is by clinging to the belief that "the cure" is just around the corner and that the newest available therapy is "the best." Recently, I was motivated to reflect on this subject upon learning that two of my patients with MS were prepared to travel across the country and invest thousands of dollars for a new vaccine heralded as having great therapeutic promise for MS. As I researched the limited literature on the vaccine, it certainly revealed appealing aspects. The strategy is to obtain a patient's T-lymphocytes that attack the nervous system's myelin, inactivate them (much like a virus would be inactivated for a vaccine), and then reintroduce them into the patient. The expectation is for the body's immune system to be geared up to combat errant lymphocytes and subdue them. So far, the procedure has been tried on a very small number of patients. Appropriate larger scale investigations are being planned.

As I visited with these two patients, it became evident that they were not put off by the very small numbers of patients for whom the vaccine had been utilized or the inherent uncertainties in the success of the procedure. For these two patients, the treatment "made sense," and they wanted to be part of it despite my reservations.

The responses offered by these two MS patients have occasioned my further reflections upon how physicians should respond to patients in such circumstances. The vaccine sounds promising and intuitively makes sense. Yet those trained in science and medicine know that a huge gulf exists between a new thesis and a therapy ultimately proven to be safe and effective. Certainly there are abundant examples in medicine of intuitive therapy that have proven futile. Two such instances in the realm of vascular disease immediately come to mind. When a patient has a completely occluded carotid artery, nothing makes more sense than to do an endarterectomy and reestablish flow. In the past, this procedure was performed on numerous patients until it was clearly established that the risks of such surgery far outweigh any prospect of benefit. Sometime thereafter, enthusiasm rose for a second, seemingly sensible surgical approach – bypassing an occluded carotid artery by connecting a branch of the superficial temporal artery to the middle cerebral artery (so-called intracranial-extracranial bypass). This surgery was performed repeatedly until a controlled study finally established that it offered no benefit to patients.

Of course, one can think of converse examples, as well, in which seemingly outlandish therapies ultimately have proven to be effective. As a resident, I well remember crazy talk about using antibiotics for ulcers. Most clinicians "knew" that this was ridiculous. The few people who championed this therapy were on the fringes of the accepted medical cannon. Twenty years later, the data about H-pylori has come along, forcing modifications in our understanding of what makes sense in ulcer treatment.

Recently, I contemplated how I might visit with the local MS support group to discuss the foregoing issues in a fashion that would prove helpful and not appear to be simply dousing the earnest hopes of those who wanted to try experimental therapies. Currently, there are various immune modulating therapies that have been demonstrated to decrease MS exacerbations and the number of new plaques visualized on the MRI over time. I have tried to understand why, when such apparently efficacious therapies exist, many patients still seem to instinctively opt for novel, unproven therapies as opposed to these more established ones. As part of this reflection I also found myself musing upon the various ineffective "remedies" that have been touted for MS during my practice lifetime. These include bee-stings, colostrum from cows' milk, removing teeth fillings, hyperbaric oxygen, snake venom, and others. Of course in the realm of "cures" the public has always been vulnerable to anecdote and "word of mouth" about new treatments. One need only look at the current enthusiasms for a wide range of herbal therapies today or to the popular and profitable patent medicines of the 19th century.

P.T. Barnum once quipped, "There's a sucker born every minute." And I suppose any of us, if we are sick enough and frightened enough, are potential "suckers" for would-be cures. I'm convinced that we can't, and probably shouldn't, dissuade our patients from clinging to hope in the nontraditional and investigative therapies. However, we should consider trying to temper the allure of the unknown simply because it is new. And I believe we should try to convince our patients not to be in the very first wave of persons who try a novel therapy, unless they are part of an appropriately structured investigational trial. I tend to remind my patients of popular treatments that have fallen by the wayside once enough was known about their risks or lack of efficacy. A decade ago, an anti-inflammatory drug was heavily marketed until it became evident that it caused aplastic anemia. More recently, a highly effective antiseizure medication was widely endorsed before its worrisome hematologic and hepatic risks became apparent. Its use in seizures has now been greatly curtailed.

The more I practice medicine, the more convinced I become that we will never have the luxury of easy answers when dealing with the complexities of illness and people's lives. Medical science always seems to court uncertainty. Presumably many of our medical truisms of today are fated to become minor footnotes to the cannon of tomorrow's scientific advancements. We must continue to work in increments to do what seems to be the best thing for patients at a given time.

Speculation

Clearly, there are many times when we don't know what those around us are thinking. I believe that is particularly true of our patients. I am struck by this fact when overhearing patients and families discussing aspects of illness, treatment, or the conduct of physicians. Oftentimes, such dialogue seems to be laced with feelings of negativity. Perhaps I inadvertently overhear these comments because unhappy people tend to talk louder than contented ones. In any event, phrases like "they don't know what's going on," "they never tell you anything," or "they never listen" are occasionally opined.

Of course, it can be very difficult to know even what our own family members and friends are thinking at times. For instance, when I was a junior in college, a good friend was my roommate for a second consecutive year. One evening, I was studying at my desk and he was standing at the sink rummaging through the medicine cabinet. Suddenly, he gave a fearsome yell, threw a tube of toothpaste onto the floor, and began stomping on it. This served to arouse my curiosity, and I made some tentative inquiry as to the cause of his behavior. When he caught his breath, he informed me that during the time we had shared a room, I had gradually been usurping the three largest shelves in the medicine cabinet for my toiletries. On the day in question, he had discovered my tube of toothpaste lying on his small fourth shelf of the cabinet. He was not contrite about the vehemency of his reaction. Indeed, in the following weeks, I believe he was quite pleased with his assertiveness. And needless to say, I did consolidate my personal items to favor a more equitable use of the medicine cabinet shelves.

From time to time, I have had similar "awakenings" in the course of my medical practice. Patients' actions or comments have suddenly emphasized a great divergence between my view of a situation and theirs. For example, I recall a middle-aged male whose evaluation confirmed a glioblastoma of the brain. I had tried to explain the nature and seriousness of this condition to him and his family. We had talked about partial surgical resection and the inability of surgery to completely remove and cure the tumor, as well as the need for subsequent radiation and chemotherapy. When the patient was nearing discharge from the hospital, I had a final conference with him and his family. As I was discussing plans for the follow-up, he suddenly interjected, "I know I have a tumor Doc, but it's not cancer is it?" I recall being shocked by the comment because, over the course of daily hospital visits, I had assumed that "tumor" and "cancer" were essentially synonymous terms. In referring to his tumor, I had intended to convey its malignant features and the essentially incurable nature of his problem. And yet, it was evident that he had been hearing something entirely different. In his mind, his brain tumor was bad, but at least it wasn't cancer.

In April of 1998, the theologian and philosopher, William F. May, visited Augustana College for an all-day workshop on health care ethics. He was at his most persuasive when talking about difficult burdens patients face in dealing with their illnesses. He has written about this topic in a work entitled *The Patient's Ordeal*.[1] One of the important points he stresses is that the patient, not the physician, shoulders the most onerous burden. This is easy for clinicians to forget when they are preoccupied, fatigued, and running behind schedule. The insecurities and frustrations that we physicians face can seem daunting and overwhelming. And yet, they pale in significance when compared to the ordeals shouldered by many of our patients.

Dr. May also speaks and writes eloquently about the importance of the physician trying to glean "the patient's story." That is, when facing diagnostic and therapeutic issues, it is not sufficient to have just the technologic expertise for treating a given condition. Rather, it is also important to enlist the patient in a conversation about the issues at hand. Only then can the caregiver begin to have some understanding of the influences affecting a patient's life. By learning the patient's values, fears, aspirations, and coping mechanisms, the physician is able to make a better judgment as to what forms of treatment/care are most appropriate for the individual. In the curriculum of the first year medical student, we educators generally begin by emphasizing the importance of the patient history. This is most appropriate. Without the benefit of such narrative, we physicians can easily lose our way in the forest of therapeutic options that may or may not be efficacious.

Sometimes, to enable the physician to understand, a jarring remark from a patient is required, almost akin to my roommate's gesture of stomping on my toothpaste. In this regard, I recall an elderly woman who, after enduring several days of aggressive diagnostic studies, asserted that her doctors "were more interested in her blood, than in her." To her mind, the physicians were focused on her electrolyte imbalances and the results of her x-rays rather than on who she was as a person and what she wanted done. At issue, of course, is not just that we physicians hear, but that we listen.

References
[1] May WF. The Patient's Ordeal. Bloomington: Indiana University Press; 1991.

By Any Other Name

Before you were listening, before most of us were paying much heed to such matters, deceptions were a regular part of medicine. It was common not to reveal the presence of cancer to a dying patient. Informed consent was implied by the patient's dutiful adherence to a doctor's learned recommendations, while patient inquiry into options and alternatives was discouraged. On rare occasions, egregious deceit was tolerated under the guise of ordinary research. Patients in the Tuskegee experiment were monitored for many years but not offered treatment for their syphilis. And of course, there were instances when placebos were used to essentially trick patients into getting better. In this seemingly remote past, if a patient's pain or other symptomatology didn't seem consistent with the perceived organic diagnosis, a "sugar pill" might be employed to assess the patient's response. If there was improvement, this was deemed evidence that the patient was faking an ailment or was the victim of so-called psychosomatic illness.

Today, we know better, or at least we hope we do. Experts generally recognize that virtually any treatment has some potential placebo effect for an individual. I have frequently heard quoted the adage that 20% of people with symptoms will benefit from a placebo. Other studies have suggested that up to 35% of patients with painful conditions experience some relief through placebo.[1] Thus, most practicing physicians now understand that if a patient is given an inert substance that is represented as treatment and the patient shows improvement, the beneficial effect noted does not necessarily mean the patient lacks organic disease. A current text on pain notes: "If about one-third of patients who have obvious physical stimuli for pain (abdominal surgery) report pain relief after a placebo injection, clearly placebos cannot be used to diagnose malingering, psychogenic pain, or any psychologic problem."[2] This contemporary understanding of placebo effect, of course, throws into disarray some previously accepted adages of clinical care.

On occasion, a physician might not even intend a placebo effect and subsequently discover the presence of one. Some years ago, I did an EEG on a patient who had somewhat bizarre spells. When I saw her a week later, she assured me that the EEG "treatment" had been totally successful and that her spells had abated. In a similar vein, I have occasionally encountered patients who felt that nerve conduction studies stimulated their nerves and relieved their symptoms. In such instances, a clinician might well ponder whether there is an ethical responsibility to undo an unintended placebo effect by insisting on brutal honesty or whether simply listening to the patient's testimonial without comment is more prudent.

Recently, the nursing staff of a local hospital questioned the practice of deliberate deception by using a placebo. The patient in question was apparently complaining of pain that seemed to her physician to be out of proportion to her disease pathology. Her physician ordered a placebo, and the nursing staff felt great uneasiness about representing a "sugar pill" as some form of valid treatment. The nursing staff brought the issue to the institutional ethics committee. It was the consensus of that group that the nursing concerns about placebo were valid and appropriate.

Contemporary bioethics literature generally concurs with the premise that the use of placebo in routine clinical care is inappropriate. The philosophic basis for concern about the placebo resides in a reverence for the principle of autonomy. Much emphasis is given to the fundamental right of patients to be intimately involved in their health care decisions. Deliberate deception of patients, or withholding important medical information, is judged to violate autonomy. Caregivers can be criticized for inappropriate paternalism when seeming to usurp a patient's need and right for truthful information. And certainly it is my sense that most patients, if appraised of the possibility, would be offended to think that their caregiver might judge their symptoms to "not be real" and give them an inert substance rather than a form of actual treatment.

For most general rules, one can posit exceptions. Perhaps in very infrequent circumstances, the use of placebo outside of a clinical trial is defensible. Most of the time, it is not. In instances in which a placebo might formerly have been used to try to determine the organicity of a patient's symptoms, it now seems more appropriate to honestly confront the individual with the caregiver's concerns and recommendations. Placebo is derived from a Latin word which means "I shall please."[3] But almost always, placebos do not please the individuals who receive them as implied treatment and later learn of this deception. A placebo by any other name is deceit. The use of placebo should not be condoned or enabled in the realm of ordinary clinical practice.

References

[1] Beauchamp TL, Childress JF. Principles of Biomedical Ethics. 3rd ed. New York: Oxford University Press; 1989.
[2] McCaffrey M, Pasero C. Pain Clinical Manual. 2nd ed. Mosby; 1999.
[3] Beauchamp and Childress.

The Physician as Hero

From the dawn of time, humans have demonstrated an instinctive affinity for the epic tale. George Lucas has skillfully recognized and nurtured this appeal in his *Star Wars* series. Like all great epics, Lucas' narratives succeed in portraying monumental struggles between the forces of good and evil.

One measure of Lucas' success is the high regard he was accorded by the renowned teacher, Joseph Campbell. For many, Campbell is best known for the series of interviews he did with Bill Moyers (subsequently published in the book, *The Power of Myth*). During his lifetime, Campbell was regarded as the preeminent authority on mythology and its relationship to modern society. He pondered the meanings of ritual and spirituality that are inextricably woven into human culture. And he loved the *Star Wars* series.

In his writing and teaching, Campbell was very interested in the concept of the hero. He believed that "the hero symbolizes our ability to control the irrational savage within us." He noted that it is the nature of the hero to have a journey and that this quest must not be for oneself but for "the wisdom and the power to serve others." The hero generally makes sacrifices to achieve this goal. Campbell talks about "a truly heroic transformation of consciousness" that takes place as the hero is subsumed into a noble enterprise. Invariably, this quest is larger than the individual who is striving for a common good.[1]

It occurs to me that Campbell's notions of heroism can be readily applied to the role of the physician. Specifically, I think that it is laudable and appropriate for practicing physicians to strive to be heroic in the performance of their duties. In many ways, the practice of medicine offers a straightforward way to act courageously. Medicine presumes self-sacrifice for the good of patients, and the medical profession can certainly provide the physician with both the wisdom and the power to be of service to others. Insofar as this is the very nature of medical practice, it may be easier for a physician to be heroic than for persons in many other occupations. The very fact that serious illness renders a patient vulnerable and dependent upon the physician may also add to the perceived lofty stature of the physician in the course of illness treatment.

The critical question, it seems to me, is whether a caregiver commits to striving for an heroic stance or becomes content with less lofty goals. At the beginning of Dickens' *David Copperfield*, a young boy wonders "whether I shall turn out to be the hero of my own life."[2] I believe this same query is appropriately pondered by physicians. While we have it in our power to conceive of our work as a noble quest, such an orientation is not an invariable component of all medical practices. It is certainly possible for a physician to emphasize the business aspects of medical practice as opposed to the service nature of it.

Unfortunately, having the possibility of heroism virtually built into the nature of medicine puts physicians at some risk of not meeting society's expectations. It seems beyond dispute that many patients and family members are unhappy with the medical profession. Sometimes these attitudes are beyond our control as people try to cope with the devastations of illness. However, I think we all hear of other instances in which the public is put off by the imperious behavior of a physician or by perceived aloofness, greed, or lack of personal concern for the patient.

One of the recurring themes in *Star Wars* has to do with the temptations that confront the powerful. The allure of the "dark side" is keen, and some warriors in *Star Wars* succumb. The physician, too, may fall victim to influences that detract from the healing mission. Debate may exist as to when this occurs. If one thinks of the physician as primarily an entrepreneur, the constraint of market forces might reasonably dominate physician behavior. On the other hand, it has been suggested by Crawshaw, et al., that medicine is "at its center, a moral enterprise grounded in a covenant of trust."[3] This formulation sounds very much like Campbell's notion of the hero who uses wisdom and power to serve others. It implies an invitation to the physician to strive for an heroic demeanor in the daily work of caregiving. Arguably, the key to both heroism and physician duty is service. It is what we do when we are at our best.

.

References

[1] Campbell J. with Moyers B. The Power of Myth. New York: Doubleday; 1988.
[2] Dickens C. David Copperfield. New York: American Library; 1962.
[3] Crawshaw et al. Patient-physician covenant. JAMA. 1995; 273:1553.

Practical Wisdom

Recently, in the company of several colleagues, I had the opportunity to reflect upon the importance of on-the-job experience in the practice of medicine. A physician finishes medical school and residency primed with the most recent scientific data and knows more about obscure pathways and the nuances of pharmacology than ever will be known again in a practice lifetime. But that's only part of the story and often not the critical theme. Rather, my fellow physicians uniformly agreed that, as they gained experience and insight over time, the practical work of diagnosis and treatment was greatly facilitated. This, I believe, is what Aristotle extolled as "practical wisdom." He noted that, in addition to the importance of the theoretical sciences, one needs understanding gleaned from doing the work. I remember, as a medical student, hearing an occasional professor elaborate on the "art" and the "science" of medicine. In my judgment, much of medicine's "art" resides in the practical wisdom born of attentive clinical experience.

In a field removed from medicine (except by analogy), my father-in-law, Francis, makes similar observations about gardening. He recalls that as a young man, eager to have a prodigious garden, he "just didn't get it" in terms of ordering his priorities for success. Each spring he would enthusiastically plant a large area, envisioning the lush produce he expected to enjoy. However, his focus would invariably become distracted by other pursuits. As a consequence of procrastination, he vividly recalls working his way through mid-summer gardens on his hands and knees in search of his prized vegetables amid the weeds. And he'd vow to be more diligent the following year.

Eventually, as he grew older, Francis learned the essence of effective gardening. He came to understand that timeliness is critical. Knowing when to use the hoe and cultivator makes all the difference. Immature plants can be uprooted if cultivating is done too early. And even with judicious cultivation, stubborn weeds still appear and require timely hoeing to prevent them from flourishing. Francis notes that if the gardener ever needs to hoe an entire garden, it is likely that the cultivating was neglected for too long. He also observes that advancing age provides the patience and perspective needed to perform these garden tasks in their appropriate sequence. The impetuousness and distractibility of youth is an impediment to orchestrating the care of the vegetable garden in optimal fashion.

Like gardening, medicine is nurtured by practical wisdom that values studied patience and perspective. These attributes assist the physician in deciding what to do and when to do it. Numerous examples from medical practice come to mind including the expanding field of complementary medicine. Clearly, the use of complementary therapies is burgeoning. In his latest study, Eisenberg notes that about 40% of the population now acknowledges using some form of complementary therapy. This percentage has increased steadily over the last decade.[1]

The physician is confronted with the difficulties of discerning which complementary therapies a given patient is using; the safety of these regimens, especially in the context of other required medical treatment; and the efficacy of various complementary therapies. Despite the enthusiasm for such therapies among the public, many physicians remain dubious and disapproving of these remedies, judging them to be ineffective. But many patients are poised to be dissatisfied with physicians who summarily reject the use of complementary therapies.

From my perspective, this is a realm where practical wisdom can be of assistance. As physicians, we need to be understanding of the personal and societal factors that impel so many millions of patients to use complementary therapies. Often, it is not judicious, or ultimately helpful, for us to summarily disparage these efforts. Rather, I think practical clinical wisdom demands that we try to accommodate patients' needs and desires into what we deem most appropriate medical treatment. As a part of these efforts, we should sufficiently investigate complementary therapies being used to ensure ourselves that patients are not at risk for obvious toxicities or drug interactions. For many patients, merely asking about complementary therapy is an indication that the physician is taking an holistic approach to their problem. And if no obvious harm is being done to a patient by complementary remedies, I believe that the physician can be tolerant of them. Herein lies the importance of physician perspective. We don't always have to agree with what our patients do. Our mandate is to try to help people. By acknowledging some patients' wishes for complementary therapies and integrating these options with conventional medical therapy, we may well be devising the best therapeutic options for these individuals.

Certainly not all clinicians exhibit the type of practical wisdom I am advocating. As with gardening, some physicians may be too focused on dramatic remedial interventions. In gardening, this type of shortsighted focus can take the form of undue enthusiasm for the year's most popular hybrids, lavish expenditure on the newest garden equipment, and premature focus upon the expected harvest. Unless the gardener does the regular work of diligently and methodically cultivating and hoeing, these expenditures and grand visions of harvest may yield disappointing results. Similarly in medicine, all of us are attracted to dramatic, decisive treatments. When we prevent a stroke with carotid endarterectomy or a heart attack with angioplasty, there is inevitably a feeling of great satisfaction for our technical and scientific prowess. However, our intimate work with patients demands more than just choosing flashy and decisive therapies. We need to know and understand our patients in order to devise the best treatments for them. In learning an individual's story, with its multi-tiered influences and motivations, it is important to focus on particulars. As Eisenberg's studies indicate, for many patients these particulars include aspects of complementary medicine.

Thus it makes sense to perceive the use of complementary therapies as opportunities to exercise practical wisdom. We need to earnestly work to understand what our patients believe and assist them in finding a suitable balance of treatment options. Often our small courtesies and compromises can yield gratifying results in the effort to assist our patients with their dreary burdens.

References
[1] Eisenberg DM, et al. Trends in alternative medicine use in the United States, 1990-1997: Results of a follow-up national survey. JAMA. 1998 Nov 11: 1569-1579.

Telephone Etiquette

The time has come, I believe, to address the controversial issue of telephone etiquette. This causes me considerable ambivalence because I believe that I am both a victim and a perpetrator of telephone disharmony. Recently, however, I suffered such an egregious impropriety (from my perspective) that I have determined to come out of the closet, so to speak, on this issue.

In the midst of a particularly chaotic day with patients, I was called out of an examination room to take a phone call from a physician. When I answered the phone, expecting to talk to the consultant, it turned out that a nurse was on the phone. I was put on hold and entertained with "elevator music." Some time later the nurse returned and ruefully informed me that her doctor had taken another call and was unavailable. She wondered if he could call me back later. This incident struck me as the proverbial last straw. The time for telephone truth and righteousness had arrived.

Clearly, the most courteous behavior is for a physician to personally place a telephone call to another colleague. In that case, a civil conversation can ensue with neither party feeling taken advantage of. Unfortunately, my experience has demonstrated that to personally place such a call to another colleague is increasingly inconvenient and time-consuming. When calling either hospitals or clinics, it has become common to experience multiple rings before the phone is finally answered. Oftentimes the voice at the other end is a recorded one listing various options and buttons to push depending on one's preference. In our office, we now have telephones that indicate the elapsed time from when a call was initiated. It is not uncommon to spend five or ten minutes "on hold" as the party being sought comes to the phone. Especially when I'm running behind, or if I am dealing with seriously ill patients or distraught families, a ten minute hiatus in order to accomplish a simple telephone conversation is a monumental affront. On the other hand, I am ambivalent about having my staff place a telephone call for me, and then trying to get me to the telephone quickly enough so that the waiting party is not aggrieved. On occasion I have bolted out of an examining room and into my office to breathlessly commence a call I probably should have initiated myself.

I see no easy solutions here. To personally place a call can be frustrating. Indeed, it is not uncommon to be holding on the phone for a time, only to learn that the party being sought is not available. On the other hand, whenever I have office staff place a call to someone, I worry that the person being called will take umbrage at being put "on hold" until I come to the phone.

Depending on the persons involved, this can easily become an "ego thing." Verbal sparring and even outright rancor can develop. The issue of who waits for whom can quickly become an issue of "pecking order." Of course, much depends on how hassled the individuals are on the day in question. If I am not seeing patients in the afternoon and am methodically reviewing charts, I might not become overly disturbed about holding on the phone for a time, as I busy myself at my desk. However, when my visit with a patient is interrupted, or if I am hurrying to complete office hours in order to get to the emergency room, the intrusion of a telephone call seems momentous. And if I perceive that my efforts are met by a patent discourtesy on the part of a caller, the ensuing conversation is destined to be strained.

As with many of the intricacies of interpersonal relationships, there are no easy answers here. I generally find myself trying to make the best of uncertain circumstances. Depending on my mood, the degree of chaos in the office, whether I am on call, and the weather, I sometimes personally place phone calls, and at other times I do not. Given the diverse factors that can influence behavior, any readers of these reflections who have received calls from me should not make damning inferences based solely upon how a given call was made.

There are extenuating circumstances in all of our lives. Hopefully, we can balance these such that we are not perpetually feeling put upon and convinced that our lot is more burdensome than that of the next person. Sometimes it may be, other times not.

Presumably, if we strive for a middle ground and consideration in our interactions with each other, things will generally work out satisfactorily. I believe that an effort to cultivate equanimity in our interactions with colleagues is desirable. On those occasions when I have been particularly irritated with a colleague over telephone unpleasantness or delays, I have not infrequently discovered that valid mitigating circumstances do exist. I suppose this boils down to little more than the Golden Rule. But with many of life's adages, a truism is easier to embrace in the abstract than on the firing line of tumultuous medical practice. The expansiveness of one's perspective seems to be key here.

Collective Conscience:
the Ethics Committee and Community

Some time ago, I was asked to visit the hospital of a medium-sized community to talk about ethics committees. This hospital had formed an ethics committee some years earlier and had watched interest and participation dwindle, particularly among physicians. In being asked to speak, it was my impression that there was a hope that I could somehow instill enthusiasm and commitment about the importance of institutional ethics committees. This struck me then and now as a big order. It has been my experience that in hospitals of any size, there frequently are a small number of people interested in, and committed to, issues of medical ethics and many more who would rather not give much thought to the topic.

Over the past 25 years, hospital ethics committees have been generally perceived as having three functions: convening to consider quandaries in patient care, education of committee members as to how to analyze and respond to ethical problems, and giving input to hospitals relative to policies and procedures with ethical impact. These are laudable objectives.

However, to meet my perceived challenge of energizing a near-dormant ethics committee, I had the insistent notion that some new emphasis was advised. And it occurred to me that an ethics committee, in principle and in fact, is fundamentally an instrument of community. That is, ethical problems seldom arise in isolation. Rather, they consistently spring up in the context of social relationships. While in the past many experts have reduced ethical problems to the application of relevant ethical principles to a given patient situation, I believe that refocusing on the dynamics of community has merit. This is not to demean the traditional patient/physician relationship. Rather, it is an assertion that our critical decisions are made in the context of communities that warrant analysis.

With virtually any hospitalized patient, three distinct but logically interrelated communities readily come to mind. First, the patient generally brings the community of family or significant others. While medicine has cherished the intimacy and confidentiality of the doctor/patient relationship, most patients, in my experience, want members of their broader community to be involved in discussions and decision making. This concept of the patient community was recently elaborated upon by Levine and Zuckerman in their article, "The Trouble with Families: Toward an Ethic of Accommodation."[1] These authors observe that "an ethic of accommodation emphasizes the need to negotiate care plans that do not compromise patients' basic interest but that recognize the capacities and limitations of family members." They also note that by focusing on human relationships, the various needs of a patient are most likely to be achieved. While many caregivers have somewhat cynically tended to view families as "trouble" standing in the way of getting things done, validation of their concerns and an emphasis on communication can help ensure that the family community serves as a resource in the treatment effort.

A second important community revolves around the health care team. Premier medicine today is virtually never done in isolation. The physician requires the support of numerous others. This is particularly true in the hospital where the patient feels the impact of numerous staff, including nursing, social work, pharmacy, and various therapists. The power of effective teamwork has recently been demonstrated to me in a multidisciplinary specialty clinic for patients with multiple sclerosis. Especially in the team meetings, following a morning of various assessments, the utility of a broad perspective of the patient's problems is evident. As a neurologist, I have considerable experience with the manifestations of MS. I am adept at various treatments, including current state-of-the-art immune modulating therapy. At each team conference I learn a great deal about our patients. The social worker may well expand my understanding of family dynamics or financial concerns. The physical therapist can help me understand certain subtleties of the patient's gait and balance problems. And the pharmacist may well provide insights into the almost mystical reliance upon various herbs and vitamins that some patients and families demonstrate. Similarly, functioning as an inter-disciplinary team, the ethics committee of an institution may serve as a paradigm example of collegial effort within the hospital. In effect, members of institutional ethics committees can help promulgate the message that the provision of medical care is necessarily a team effort.

A third community of note involves the sometimes nebulous character of institutions themselves. Hospitals, like other organizations, have a history and a culture. A not-for-profit hospital might readily cite its mission statement as a guide to its activities. But I think that it is important to recognize that a hospital culture is invariably in flux and that ethics committee members can serve as an important resource to an institution. Specifically, the committee can regularly ponder whether hospital policies and initiatives are, in fact, consistent with the mission statement. While some executives of an institution may view this role as potentially stirring up controversy, it seems possible to me that ethics committee members and hospital executives can, in fact, champion regular dialogue as a means of continued quality improvement for an institution. Perhaps one way to set the stage for such conversation is to arrange for an institution's executive management and members of the ethics committee to jointly attend formal educational sessions dealing with business ethics.

My belief is that specific emphasis on the communal nature of ethical decision making can prove to be useful and invigorating for an ethics committee. While much traditional medical ethics education has focused on the use of basic ethical principles applied to the doctor/patient relationship, a broader perspective can be helpful. When emphasis is given to seeing the patient in the context of his or her story, invariably community roles are brought forward. Instead of seeing the patient as an isolated and sometimes alienated individual, a person with illness is more properly seen in the context of an evolving life story. Family relationships may be an incredible source of support, or they may be destructive. The fears, misconceptions, and hopes that patients and companions bring to the milieu of illness care should be recognized. Ethics committee members can hone their clinical skills by considering actual patient cases or fictional narratives in the important light of contextual influences. Such an emphasis can effectively demonstrate that ethical principles are not technical tools to be dispassionately wielded in the abstract but rather instruments to be reverently brought to the particulars of patients' lives.

In summary, an ethics committee should see itself as validating and promoting the integrated communities surrounding the patient, the caregivers, and the institution. Such a focus on community relationships can help define the mission of ethics committees. As individuals and committee members, we never have all the answers. But collective conscience can sometimes help show us the way.

References

[1] Levine C, Zuckerman C. The Trouble with Families: Toward an Ethic of Accommodation. Annals of Internal Medicine. 1999 Jan 15:148-152.

On Medical Challenges and Monet

In the fall of 1995, my wife and I joined friends in Chicago to view the Claude Monet collection at the Art Institute. This much acclaimed exhibit was spectacular. It included 159 pieces, making it the largest retrospective of Monet's work ever assembled. Enthusiasm for this show reached a fevered pitch, and, in the final weeks of the exhibit, tickets for admittance were sold out.

The paintings were, of course, intriguing and sometimes breathtaking. Besides the works themselves, two things in particular interested me. First, I was fascinated by the apparent ease and expertise that the Art Institute of Chicago demonstrated in accommodating the hoards of visitors to the exhibit. An estimated 800 people an hour worked their way through the collection. While there were notable queues to tolerate and necessary jostling to get close to each painting, people generally seemed patiently enthusiastic for the adventure. Simply watching the diverse spectators proved to be of considerable interest.

A second aspect that impressed me was the history of Monet's painting career. Specifically, I was intrigued to learn of the difficulties and occasional dangers that attended his painting. Somehow this seemed particularly surprising given the generally serene settings captured in his impressionistic landscapes. In fact, it appears that Monet endured notable hardship in his quest to find the most suitable subjects. For instance, in 1883, he apparently scaled a vertical cliff in order to reach an isolated beach with a promising perspective. Unfortunately, he miscalculated the incoming tide, was thrown against the cliff, and lost his painting equipment. In the following year, Monet is described as painting in the midst of a hail storm. And in 1887 he was observed returning from an outing of painting "swathed in three overcoats...his face half-frozen" after being out in the elements to study some aspect of snow.[1]

Such anecdotes made me think about how little we may know of the tribulations and risks faced by professions other than our own. Certainly my image of an artist generally has involved the notion of a languid pose at a comfortable easel. By extension, I suspect that most nonmedical people have little appreciation for the complexity and challenge of doing medicine well. From a distance, medicine might easily appear to be a lucrative and straightforward enterprise, with no heavy lifting. Whereas those ensconced in the trenches of health care understand that being a good physician is neither easy nor straightforward.

Once, while I was teaching undergraduate students, I elaborated on this issue. One of the students wondered, somewhat indignantly, why physicians are always late. That day had proven to be a good case in point for me and I expounded on it at some length to the class. My schedule had included a number of established patients, all with clearly defined problems. I had begun my morning in the office precisely on time. However the second appointment, an anticipated quick follow-up for Parkinson's disease, proved to be a tumultuous session dealing with the patient's anger and depression about her disease. The yarn of interpersonal interaction in her family was unraveling, and she was desperate for someone to listen and assist her. Instead of a 15 minute follow-up, I spent almost an hour with her and still left with the feeling that she needed more time. Obviously, my schedule for the remainder of the morning, and indeed the afternoon, was significantly impacted. I tried to explain to the students that the urgency of being present to a patient in need frequently must take precedence over the niceties of scheduling.

Clearly, this experience is not unique or unusual. It is also not uncommon for us to have to confront fearful tragedies as a result of illness and death. Frequently we caregivers deal with patients and families at their worst as they struggle with the grim realities of disease and the anger and frustration which can attend it. Sometimes we take physical risks, as in dealing with patients harboring infectious diseases. Often, if we give our patients as much of our time as they require, our own family time and outside interests are necessarily constrained.

What counts, in the end, is how successful the physician and the artist are in achieving their ideals. Monet certainly did not have to scale a vertical cliff and risk unpredictable tides in order to be acclaimed. But the perfectionist in him must have demanded that he seek a certain difficult perspective in the time and space he was allotted. Similarly, physicians can easily burden themselves with time-consuming interactions and emotional tumult if willing to practice their art as they best perceive it. As with Monet, perfection in medicine may well demand focus and rigor well beyond the view of the casual observer.

References
[1] The Art Institute of Chicago's brochure for Claude Monet 1840-1926. 1995 July 22-Nov 26.

On Metaphor

An integral part of our humanity seems to be the ability to think and speak in metaphor. We do it all the time. A functional definition of metaphor, blended from various sources, is "a figure of speech comparing essentially unlike things." We use metaphor when we talk of the "war on drugs" or "computer memory."

From the standpoint of clinical care, a metaphor might prove either helpful or counterproductive. For instance, physicians are sometimes accused of "playing God" when difficult treatment (or often non-treatment) decisions are made. The derogatory implication of this metaphor is that the physician is somehow usurping an action properly left to the Deity. Examples of "playing God" might include stopping a ventilator of a comatose 70 year old with massive brain hemorrhage and virtually no chance of meaningful recovery or stopping tube feedings in the case of a patient in a permanent vegetative state, such as the late Nancy Cruzan. Physicians make such difficult decisions all the time. These actions may be medically and ethically appropriate, or not, depending on complex variables. The use of the term "playing God" may obfuscate, rather than clarify, such unavoidable decision making that falls to the lot of the physician. The pervasiveness of this metaphor is reflected in frequent literary references to the physician acting in a godlike capacity. For example, in Marcia Lynch's poem about breast cancer she notes, "you are the Gods I believed in as a child. I prayed you to pull magic out of your black leather bags to waive away the rattling in my bones."[1] Another example is Anne Sexton's poem which notes that doctors "are not Gods, though they would like to be; they are only a human trying to fix up a human. Many humans die."[2]

Some years ago, the USD School of Medicine held an all-day seminar entitled, "AIDS: Today's Epidemic." In preparation for this event, I read two books – *AIDS and Its Metaphors* by Susan Sontag[3] and *The Promise of Rest* by Reynolds Price.[4] Sontag has long argued that society does a grave disservice to patients with illness by metaphorically labeling diseases. She points out that in past decades cancer was viewed with revulsion, while tuberculosis was perceived with some sentimentality. She contends that the "metaphoric trappings that deform the experience of having cancer have very real consequences: they inhibit people from seeking treatment early enough..." Similarly, she notes that AIDS is often thought of metaphorically. Instead of being simply a devastating viral infection, it is perceived in some circles as being divine retribution for unacceptable behavior. Sontag argues that physicians and society burdened patients by foisting such metaphorical baggage onto their shoulders in addition to the already devastating weight of serious disease.

In Price's novel, he similarly alludes to metaphor. Wade, the protagonist, is dying of AIDS. His friend comments that "the power deep in him finally thrust him out in the path of the cruelest plague in 600 years. I don't need to tell this smart a crowd the lowdown truth – that when people say this curse was sent by Fate to punish a special brand of human, we ought to ask – right back in their teeth – whether they think leukemia is sent to punish the millions of children that die of it everywhere..."[4]

Surely not all metaphor is suspect, however. We may also use such images to enhance and ennoble our profession. The following brief bit of poetry by Larry Schafer, M.D. is an elegant example:

> Prehensile grasp
> digital apposition
> finger extended
> to touch the face of God.

This piece evokes the image of Michelangelo and the Sistine Chapel, where a bearded God extends a finger to touch the outstretched hand of a human being. One might argue that far from serving up the negative connotations imputed by the term "playing God," Dr. Schafer's poem can be construed to

119

illustrate humankind's empowerment and challenge to reach beyond the mundane world to heightened potentials. Perhaps the poetic example (and Michelangelo's visual one) of reaching out, might signify the awesome ability of humanity to move beyond individual priorities and to rationally embrace the burden of caring for one another. At least I have chosen to think of Schafer's poem in this fashion as I have been reflecting on our obligations to care for persons with HIV/AIDS. The various speakers at the medical school seminar on AIDS articulated the need for all physicians to be sufficiently knowledgeable about HIV disease to appropriately include it in the differential diagnosis of a myriad of clinical conditions. The faculty of this seminar quietly demonstrated by their own attitudes and clinical vignettes their belief that physicians have an obligation to care for all persons with disease, regardless of the etiology and social nuances.

It seems to me that, as physicians, we must strive ardently to develop a broad and encompassing world view rather than a mean-spirited and constricted one. In our work, we inevitably will come in contact with patients whose social mores, religious beliefs, and personalities differ from our own. Especially since our professional practices expose us to the intimate details of patient and family life, we are often fated to deal with disturbing realities. Arguably, one of our critical duties as physicians is to try to instill in ourselves and our colleagues the notion that we must be broadminded and compassionate rather than condemning and exclusionary. By striving for a nonjudgmental attitude as we deal with patients, we in no way condone self-destructive behaviors that may lead to HIV infection such as IV drug usage or multiple sexual partners. Similarly, we grieve the implications of a 20 year old motorcycle rider lying comatose in an ICU for lack of a helmet; or a 55 year old with a 40 year history of cigarette smoking that has resulted in a lung tumor. Ideally, we offer treatment for the people who present to us without discrimination based on the etiology of a malady. Necessarily, this requires that caregivers work to see patients as individuals in need of assistance, regardless of their personal beliefs and life-styles.

In the Marcia Lynch poem I previously quoted, she states, "In this disease there is no sin." [1] Patients always have, and always will, make ill-advised life-style decisions. We can be angry at this reality, but as caring physicians we cannot let our attitudes translate into a punitive approach to the patient once disease has taken hold. In the grim world of illness and death, there is enough tragedy and pain. We do not want to add to the patient's burden by recrimination and judgmental metaphor. While we cannot always ameliorate a patient's problems, we certainly must strive to not add to their woes.

References

[1] Lynch M. Peau D'Orange. In: Jon Mukand, ed. Sutured Words. Aviva Press; 1987.

[2] Sexton, A. Doctors. In: Jon Mukand, ed. Sutured Words. Aviva Press; 1987.

[3] Sontag S. Illness as Metaphor and AIDS and Its Metaphors. New York: Doubleday; 1977, 1988.

[4] Price R. The Promise of Rest. New York: Scribner 1995.

Dealing with Devastation

Often my Uncle Don gazes upon me from his framed vantage point. He has been doing that forever, or at least for the over fifty years that I have been able to consciously look back at him. He seems to have the jaunty confidence of a twenty-something young man on the verge of seizing his destiny. His hair is roguishly combed back and his white silk scarf is perfectly positioned over the collar of his aviator's jacket. As a child, and indeed even as an adolescent, I dreamed of him returning from the ambiguous status of "missing in action." I pictured how it would be to see him strolling down the lane toward my grandparents' home with the same easy smile that was frozen in his photograph. In that dramatic way, I dreamed, he would dispel my grandparents' smoldering anguish at having lost their only son in World War II combat, and he would infuse happiness into our family circle.

Of course he never came, and in truth, I grew weary of his unblinking gaze upon me. After my grandmother died, the grandchildren convened at her home to decide how to disperse or discard her life's mementos, accumulated in the home she occupied for almost eighty years of her adult life. I was vaguely surprised when my wife chose to bring home a number of old portraits, including that of my Uncle Don. Indeed, at first I was almost uneasy having him stare back at me in my own home. It is remarkable to think that I am now almost twice the age of this mysterious fellow who flew off to the South Pacific, never to return.

I believe that part of the reason I have been reflecting upon Uncle Don is because of my general brooding upon the devastating events that can occur in people's lives. Some years ago, I treated a young woman about Uncle Don's age when he was photographed. A tragic gymnastic accident resulted in a severe compression fracture of a thoracic vertebra. Presumably, her fall from the uneven bars occurred with the same type of devastating swiftness with which my uncle's plane dropped from the sky and cleaved the Pacific Ocean.

To some extent, all of my grandparents' long lives after Don's accident were a form of attempted rehabilitation from the effects of their loss. Similarly, there is a part of my young patient and her family that will always be in rehabilitation, even as she makes some recovery.

One of the most noble things we do in medicine is to effectively care for those who sustain these types of personal devastations in their lives. For the past fifteen years or so I have been involved in helping teach a class on caring to undergraduate students at Augustana College. Certainly in life and in literature, one can find many examples of caring behavior. Yet, I continue to find it difficult to define what caring means. In this regard, caring may be like such entities as justice, love, and art in that we all can cite examples (or lack) of these concepts, but might struggle at arriving at a precise definition.

I believe that a superb demonstration of caring is found in Leo Tolstoy's short novel, *The Death of Ivan Ilych*.[1] During the latter stages of Ivan's terminal illness, his steward, Gerasim, serves a nursing role for Ivan. He does "what has to be done" in terms of striving to make Ivan comfortable. Gerasim massages Ivan's legs, assists him with his bodily wastes, and serves as Ivan's companion. Gerasim's caring behavior stands in stark contrast to the detachment and reserve that Ivan's family and friends exhibit toward him.

In the course of these reflections, I seem to have ranged a considerable distance from the uncle I never knew to a young patient who is almost daily before me as a focus of medical concern and empathy. Perhaps I initially juxtaposed their two lives because I was struck by the swift devastation that can befall any of us, including the young, and by the almost boundless need for care and compassion in such situations. It is always difficult to move beyond the pain of permanent loss. To some extent, I believe my grandparents continued to struggle with this issue throughout their long lives. As a bystander, a generation removed, I still ponder "what might have been" as I gaze upon my uncle's photograph. Similarly, my young gymnast patient and her family must continue to ponder the whimsy of fate and to quail at unknown prospects for the future.

In my opinion, one of the greatest literary allegories about human happenstance and catastrophe is Thornton Wilder's book, *The Bridge of San Luis Rey*.[2] This work studies the lives of five unfortunate individuals who happened to be on the bridge the day it collapses, plunging them to their deaths. In the last sentence of the book, Wilder says: "There is a land of the living and a land of the dead and the bridge is love, the only survival, the only meaning." All of us, of course, constitute the ranks of current survivors as we deal with the death or impairments of loved ones or with our own physical assaults. The idea that love can help mitigate these traumas and unite us is powerful. The key, perhaps, is how that love is made manifest. In my grandparents' case, they compensated for their tragic loss with devotion to their grandchildren. Gerasim served by his steady presence and an attitude that no effort for a dying patient was too menial or trivial to perform. My gymnast patient's circle of family and friends and caregivers have been able to effectively collaborate to ease her suffering and help her cope with major disability. Love is not a term we use readily in the clinical realm. However, it clearly has everything to do with caring and survival and meaning.

References

[1] Tolstoy L..The Death of Ivan Ilych and Other Stories. New York: The New American Library; 1960.

[2] Wilder T. The Bridge of San Luis Rey. New York: Washington Square Press; 1939.

When Shouldn't We Treat?

Years ago, I was visiting the home of a colleague. He noted that his young daughter was complaining of her ears hurting. He had looked at them and thought they appeared fine, but he wanted my opinion. Dutifully, I too attempted to study the tympanic membranes of the somewhat uncooperative daughter. As I recall, I shrugged and said her ears didn't look too bad to me either. Later that evening, her parents rushed their daughter to an emergency room as the ear symptoms worsened. She proved to have a significant otitis media. While my friend subsequently joked about our diagnostic acumen in pediatrics, his experience is certainly a cautionary tale. There are times when a physician should not treat immediate family members.

This topic of treating one's own family was discussed at an institutional ethics committee meeting I recently attended. The group's comments were intriguing. A number of clinicians distinguished between engaging in fairly routine care for a family member as opposed to participating in a more invasive intervention. Two physicians noted that, in the past, they had taken a throat swab of their children to check for streptococcus. Both physicians acknowledged that, if the strep screen was positive, they proceeded to initiate antibiotics. Their rationalization in doing this was to avoid pressing their already busy colleagues into providing a routine intervention. Another physician noted that while he might obtain a throat swab, he would ask another physician to call in the prescription.

As the discussion progressed, it became evident that many of the participants were aware of times when a physician treated family members. One example cited was the practice of a physician delivering his own baby (generally with a colleague skilled in obstetrics in attendance). Another participant noted that a local physician had performed an endoscopic procedure on an immediate family member. Still another clinician volunteered that she had been involved in the care of a patient whose family member, a physician, had actually changed some of the hospital orders of the attending physician.

In the current Code of Medical Ethics, the AMA has specifically addressed such issues: "Physicians generally should not treat themselves or members of their immediate families. Professional objectivity may be compromised when an immediate family member or the physician is the patient; the physician's personal feelings may unduly influence his or her professional medical judgment, thereby interfering with the care being delivered."[1]

Sometimes moving from actual cases to a theoretical one can be helpful. One of the committee members posed the question of whether a physician father of a 16 year old girl should undertake to investigate her abdominal pain. Would he be sufficiently objective to consider all diagnostic possibilities? The AMA publication notes: "Physicians may fail to probe sensitive areas when taking the medical history or may fail to perform intimate parts of the physical examination. Similarly, patients may feel uncomfortable disclosing sensitive information or undergoing an intimate examination when the physician is an immediate family member. This discomfort is particularly the case when the patient is a minor child..."[2]

As with most of the complex psychosocial and ethical issues that confront us, there probably is no absolute standard or single dictum that should govern all physician behavior with respect to treating immediate family members. There are many variables. A therapeutic relationship that might seem ill-advised in a large city, where multiple physicians reside, might be the best or only reasonable option in a very small community with a single caregiver. In response to such complexities, the ethics committee was not eager to suggest that its hospital absolutely proscribe all instances of physicians treating immediate family members. On the other hand, there was unanimous agreement from the diverse group comprising the ethics committee that the health care community benefits from a critical consideration of these issues. As medical professionals, as well as members of society as a whole, it seems we almost never go wrong when we encourage earnest, thoughtful discussion.

Our professional judgments should be grounded in sound values. That is the essence of bioethics. Our judgments and actions should also conform to common sense. It seems likely that there will be times when many of us offer a minor medical intervention for an immediate family member. On the other hand, reflection on this topic should generally make us very cautious about the potential perils and pitfalls of such treatment. I believe most of us would agree that, as a general rule, a trusted colleague is in a better position to treat one of our family members than we ourselves are. During the course of our ethics committee discussion, one pediatrician recalled that early in his married life he told his wife that their children needed a smarter physician than he to provide appropriate care for them. From my perspective, his statement was mainly hyperbole. I've known him for many years and have great respect for his professional competence and compassion. But I am not at all surprised that as a young physician he firmly resisted treating his own children. He was being a good father. The roles we physicians are called upon to play are complex and mutable. We are highly motivated to be of use. Constantly we must remind ourselves what to do, as well as what not to do.

References

[1] American Medical Association. Code of Medical Ethics: Current Opinions with Annotations. AMA Press; 2002.
[2] Ibid.

Lessons from the Windmill

In some ways, Don Quixote has given windmills a bad name. With his indefatigable persistence at tilting toward them, windmills have (at least in some eyes) taken on the character of the imaginary or improbable. However, having one of my own, I see the windmill metaphorically but in a very different light from the Quixote perspective.

The first step in my enlightenment took place upon obtaining an old, but still functioning windmill. While sleek, new wind generators undoubtedly offer greater utility, I felt the need for an old original. It is somewhat rusted, has several memorial bullet holes through the blades, and is dented in places. But it responds beautifully to the wind. Usually, it is only at dawn that the windmill rests silently. During most days, even in a fragile breeze, it dutifully functions.

Before my infatuation with the windmill, I envisioned the wind more or less coming as a uniform force from some direction. The windmill, however, demonstrates a more complicated truth. In a steady breeze, it is almost continuously rotating in adjustment. With the tail extended to best direct the blades into a shifting breeze, the head of the windmill methodically and irregularly swivels back and forth to best advantage. And in the fiercest of winds, the tail competently folds parallel to the spinning blades, causing them to briefly lock, catch their breath, and then resume their mission of spinning in response to the wind.

This process of ongoing responsiveness and adjustment has tempted me to fashion a comparison between the windmill and medicine. The windmill's constant vigilance to the presence of wind and its skilled ability to cope with everything from tentative spurts that only flutter the leaves to a howling storm that bends flag poles, can certainly resemble the resourceful physician. In the clinical realm, one of the greatest challenges is to move from mundane, and sometimes almost trivial, afflictions to the woes of catastrophic illness. The clinician, like the sturdy windmill, must regularly adapt to both.

However, a study of the windmill's function permits an even more refined comparison. It is not sufficient for the windmill to simply adapt to variable wind speeds any more than it is for the physician to premise the nature of interaction with a patient solely on whatever type of illness the patient has. The most informative view of the windmill takes account not only of the prevailing wind direction, but also of the constant shifting of the wind. In fact, even while the blades are spinning, the tail is ceaselessly rotating the windmill head back and forth to best confront the breeze. And herein lies a most apt comparison with clinical medicine. The directions in which our patients' lives move are no more static and predictable than is the wind. Patients' fears, aspirations, family pressures, and coping mechanisms always demand individually tailored responses. Thus a given diagnosis, such as stroke, does not imply a nearly identical condition in every patient. For one person, stroke might be a minor inconvenience to be overcome. For another, it may serve as a harsh glimpse of mortality. For still another, a stroke may serve as an impetus for a family coming together, or breaking apart. Like the adaptable windmill, the physician must remain vigilant to the subtle nuances of disease in some patients, as well as the staggering burdens that obviously exist for others.

There is debate as to how best to prepare the physician to perceive these variabilities and complexities in human lives. An emphasis on narrative can serve to highlight the necessary reciprocity that exists between patient and caregiver. Rita Charon, who has long championed the importance of attentive focus upon stories of illness, notes that narrative competence includes "an awareness of the ethical complexity of the relationship between teller and listener, a relationship marked by duty toward privileged knowledge and gratitude for being heard."[1]

Recently, I heard a woman telling about her husband's experience with physicians. After her husband's doctor of many years retired, her spouse went for an initial visit to a young physician who was assuming his care. As part of a detailed history, the new physician asked about the unconventional remedies the patient was using. The husband ruefully acknowledged taking a nightly shot of gin and some raisins because he'd heard of the salutary health benefits of this regimen. He had never told his prior physician of this habit, and indeed his wife was unaware of it as well. Both the patient and his wife were very impressed by the physician's thoroughness and concern in specifically eliciting this information.

Learning about patients' whims and beliefs is not merely tilting at windmills in a quixotic sense. Rather, such focused attention can heighten empathy and understanding. Sometimes, of course, the behaviors and beliefs of a patient may appear opaque and inexplicable. And sometimes clinical focus on the intimacies of a patient's narrative can seem akin to watching a finely tuned windmill in action. That is, such observation can be deeply satisfying even without fully understanding the intricacies of windmill functioning or the atmospheric forces responsible for waxing and waning wind speed. Effective illness care demands focused attentiveness and a willingness to embrace the unpredictable in an effort to honor the idiosyncrasies of the human spirit.

References
[1] Charon R. Narrative and Medicine. New England Journal of Medicine. 2004 Feb 26; 862-3.

Regrets

All of us, I suspect, deal with gnawing regret from time to time. These feelings may be prompted by an appointment or opportunity missed, or from a more grievous loss such as the untimely death of a loved one. Inevitably as we deal with the loss, we repeatedly ask ourselves "what if things could have been different...."

Last Christmas, our family drove to central Minnesota to be with my wife's parents and some of her siblings. Although this was a long one day trip, we had an enjoyable visit. As we were leaving in the late afternoon, I fleetingly thought about going home "the long way" and surprising my sister and her large family at what I imagined would be their Christmas evening meal. But I opted not to make that impulsive change in our plans, arguing to myself that such a detour would significantly prolong our trip. During the drive home that evening and the next day, I continued to regret not having made the surprise visit. I believe my sister would have been very pleased. Christmas day is one of the rare occasions when it would have been possible to see her entire family assembled together.

My Christmas day regrets certainly pale in significance to grieving and loss that many of my patients and their families express. Indeed, I am often struck by the diverse ways in which people handle regret and loss. Recently, I encountered two literary works with characters that deal with life's losses using the metaphor of the combing or braiding of hair. Given the thinness and unruliness of my own hair, these narrative images at first seemed somewhat dubious to me. Upon dispassionate reflection, I continue to believe that this particular metaphor is very effective indeed.

Michael Dorris ends his powerful novel *A Yellow Raft in Blue Water* with the image of an elderly woman braiding her hair. This novel talks about the intersection of her life with those of her daughter and granddaughter. The grandmother is clearly in a time of emotional upheaval, and as she sits down she instinctively begins to work with her hair. She experiences "the rhythm of three strands, the whispers of coming and going, of twisting and tying and bending, of catching and of letting go, of braiding."[1]

In his short story, "Imagine a Woman," author Richard Selzer employs a somewhat similar context for his protagonist, a young woman dying of AIDS. She reflects as follows: "combing my hair (the one part of me that is thriving, it has grown very long), combing and combing with long, slow strokes, combing out the pain. I read somewhere that the women of Sparta sat in the moonlight combing their hair until their sorrows went away. It works. I fell asleep while combing...."[2]

Both of these literary characters are coping with the anguish of loss. Fictional narratives are especially compelling when they conform to our personal experiences. One of the aspects of my medical practice that most amazes me is how patients and families handle the brutal intrusions of illness and loss that can disrupt their lives. It seems to me that acts of caring, sometimes so subtle as to seem inconsequential, are what sustain people. All of us are fortunate when we have opportunities for caring interaction and seize upon them. The Christmas holiday is an apt time to reflect on the power each of us has to enrich the lives of others. But such opportunities present themselves repeatedly in everyday life. And certainly our ability to positively impact on the lives of others is potentially enhanced when we assume the role of caregiver.

When we fall short of our expectations of ourselves, we should feel disappointed. The thorn of regret should prod us to do things differently in the future. My sister and her family weren't expecting us last Christmas, and I wasn't obligated to pay a surprise visit. Yet I wish I had made the effort. A surprise visit would have been just the right thing. To paraphrase Dorris' earlier quotation, some of our comings and goings, our catching and letting go, are discretionary. Some are beyond our control. If regrets of the past prompt us to more aggressively seize opportunities for caring, so much the better. We shouldn't be too hard on ourselves, but we shouldn't be too easy either.

References

[1] Dorris, M. A Yellow Raft in Blue Water. New York: Warner; 1988.
[2] Selzer R. Imagine a Woman. In: The Doctor Stories. New York: Picador; 1998.

Recognition: The Gift Outright

Mary closed the door behind her as she entered the room and approached the elderly woman. She was sitting in sunlight, wheelchair positioned by the window. Most days her conversations with Mary were limited to answers regarding meal preferences and various discomforts. It was not clear whether she remembered Mary from one visit to the next. But on this particular day the old woman's demeanor suggested an atypical intent. Looking straight at Mary she announced "I know that you're you." She reached out to the window ledge and picked up one of the greeting cards lined up there. She turned it over in her hands, looking from the card to Mary and back again. For the first time the old woman seemed to make the connection between the holiday cards she'd been periodically receiving and Mary's weekly visits to her. Ever so briefly, the veil of her dementia seemed to be lifted, permitting unaccustomed insight. Ever so briefly, she hinted at a gratitude that mostly eluded her ability to express.

A gift can provoke unpredictable responses in both the receiver and the giver. Both can be nourished by the exchange. In his poem "The Gift Outright ," Robert Frost ponders the possibility of being given a gift whose potential far exceeds first appearances. Reflecting on the magnificent future destined to unfold for the United States of America Frost proclaims: "To the land vaguely realizing westward... Such as she was, such as she would become." [1]

Last year, as Christmas approached, Kingsley and his wife presented me with a "gift outright" when I least expected it. I had cared for Kingsley years earlier after he broke his neck. For weeks he suffered the burden of a halo brace for his neck and various other medical complications. His extremities were weak from a spinal cord injury, and he was further restricted by virtue of chronic ankylosing spondylitis. He and his wife came to the office frequently as we sorted through his problems, those that could be remedied and those that persisted.

134

The intervals between our visits gradually increased and eventually Kingsley ceased coming to my office.

Some four years after I last saw him, I was surprised to be hailed in a hospital corridor by Kingsley's wife. She indicated that he was again in the hospital and she was quite certain that he would like me to visit. He was suffering various medical maladies now, ones that did not require my intervention. Over the next week or two I periodically encountered Kingsley and his wife in the hospital, and they always seemed happy to visit.

Some months thereafter, while in a different community hospital, I again encountered Kingsley. This time he was sitting in a wheelchair in the physical therapy department. Despite his troubles, he seemed both stoic and cheerful. The following day, Kingsley's wife called my office requesting that I again stop by his hospital room. When I arrived, she presented me with what seemed to be several pounds of frozen lefse and a holiday card. She said that they just wanted to thank me for all I had done for Kingsley over the years. The card contained a gift certificate.

On reflection, it seems to me that there are a number of "gifts outright" in these two anecdotes. When the elderly lady with dementia told Mary "I know that you're you," she was clearly signaling gratitude for the attention that had been bestowed on her. And Mary was most appreciative of this unanticipated insight. Similarly, encounters with Kingsley were rewarding. I was delighted and amazed to see that Kingsley, now 81 years old, was still as mentally sharp and wry as I remembered him a decade earlier. His reappearance reminded me of a Ted Kooser poem entitled "The Very Old ." Kooser begins with the observation that "The very old are forever hurting themselves... falling loosely as trees and breaking their hips with muffled explosions of bone..." They then seem to disappear for long periods of time before "We see them again, first one and then another... perennial, checking their gauges for rain."[2] Kingsley's penchant for suddenly appearing at unexpected times evokes a sense of Kooser's "perennial"—a recurrent gift. And I suspect that Kingsley and his wife viewed my visits with them as a gift of sorts. If so, I believe I derived as much pleasure from these encounters as they did, and I was moved by their holiday gifts to me.

To return to Frost's poem, I suppose none of us fully comprehend the implications of the gifts we give, whether they be material ones or gifts of our time and talents. Gift giving, by its nature, can perpetuate itself, moving from an initial opportunity to the next and the next. Frost's poem can be a metaphor for this ripple effect as he reflects on promises yet to unfold. The process of becoming is an important part of our shared humanity. To give and to receive is to celebrate who we are and who we may become.

References

[1] Frost R. The Gift Outright In: Latham EC, editor. The Poetry of Robert Frost. New York: Holt, Rinehart & Winston; 1969.

[2] Kooser T. The Very Old . In: Sure Signs; New and Selected Poems. Pittsburgh: University of Pittsburgh Press, 1980.

In Another Time

"All the influences were lined up waiting for me. I was born, and there they were to form me, which is why I tell you more of them than of myself." [1] So speaks Augie March, the protagonist of Saul Bellow's famous novel, as he thinks back on his life. Like Augie, we are all sustained by the influences in our lives and our memory of them. They are part of us, coloring our perceptions and interactions. For my father-in-law, Francis, there appears to be a mostly comfortable continuum of influences that stretches from his boyhood to the present, his 81st year. Francis can nimbly summon the memory of such influences into stories that are true or should be.

For Francis, Josie Henkemeyer was such an influence. Francis first recalls meeting Josie upon leaving the breakfast table with the customary impatience of an eight year old and wandering into the basement. There Francis was surprised to encounter Josie combing his sparse hair with a scrub brush. At that time, Josie worked for Francis' father and had apparently been invited to breakfast. He had gone into the basement to spruce himself up before appearing at the dining table. Josie was fastidious and a proper subject for a young boy's observations. While working at a construction site, Josie predictably ended each noontime meal by removing his false teeth and cleansing his mouth with coffee from his thermos.

Francis had plenty of opportunity to observe Josie and to learn from him. Josie did carpentry with both Francis' grandfather and father. As an old man, Josie also worked for Francis' construction business as well. Over all this time, Josie served as a mentor of the subtleties of carpentry and as a foil to a changing world. Josie believed that a carpenter should never say "good enough." Proper measuring was critical. If a wall was commenced 1/16 inch shy, the discrepancy would grow to an inch at the other end of the room. As he grew older, Josie's commitment to impeccable measurements became something of a burden. In his late 70's, when he was still doing some finish carpentry, Josie would measure, then remeasure, then measure again. Eventually, his scruples for proper measurement began to seriously intrude upon his efficiency as a carpenter.

Over the years, Francis has so frequently recalled stories about Josie that I have almost come to believe I knew him. Josie was a master at certain tasks such as sharpening a saw by properly setting the teeth. Generally, Josie didn't just cut a board in two, but would saw to the unmistakable cadence of the jingle "Shave and a haircut — two bits." Even from a distance, Francis recalls, one could pick out Josie coming to a new worksite in the morning. He would remove his white pine workbench from the back of his Model A and sling it over his right shoulder. He had customized the bench for his specific needs. It had a rail that ran its length so that Josie could set a door on the rail and then clamp it to the bench with a small, attached vise. Held in that position he could plane the edge of the door to fit the jam and could mortice the hinges. A trough at the bottom of the bench served to hold tools such as his rule and bevel square while he was working. The workbench also served as a seat for the noontime meal, and Josie could stand on it to do work that was above his comfortable reach.

It is interesting to appreciate the impact that early influences have on an individual. Like Josie, Francis now rarely uses a handsaw without breaking into the cadence that Josie employed. And Francis became an expert at sharpening saws after learning from Josie how critical a properly prepared saw is to carpentry.

I have frequently urged Francis to retell stories of Josie, particularly of his idiosyncrasies. As a workday progressed, the right side of Josie's nose became increasingly black. He regularly rubbed nails along his nose, knowing that skin oil made them easier to pound. Josie rarely picked something up without first licking his right thumb. His manner of holding a cigarette was both peculiar and unique. The cigarette was always positioned between his second and third fingers and brought to his lips with his hand facing outward. Indeed that posture was so distinctive, and has been described to us so many times, that a member of our family need only hold up a hand in this fashion to signal that something triggered a memory of Josie.

One story that Francis particularly enjoys took place when Francis was working for his father along with Josie. The owner of the home being built invited the three carpenters to dinner at a formal supper club in Marshall, Minnesota. None of the crew had ever dined in such fashion. At the supper club, everyone ordered steaks. Presently a waiter officiously arrived with a large steak which he placed in front of Josie. Josie picked up his knife and fork, judiciously looked around at his three companions at the table, and then cut his steak into four parts, ready to share. He was a humble man and sure there was enough steak on his plate for everyone. Just as he was commencing to pass his plate around the table, the waiter returned with the rest of the meals and set a plate before each man. Francis recalls that Josie was more or less nonplussed by the incident but was able to finish all four pieces of steak on his plate!

It is intriguing for me to reflect upon Josie's legacy as it has been perpetuated in Francis' reflections. Like all of us, Francis has had many influences that helped shape his life. Some were momentous events and some were almost incidental encounters. But all contributed to the formation of the energetic and creative person Francis became. Presumably, many influences in one's life remain forgotten and unacknowledged. But fortunately, our recollections and stories often enable us to summon prior influences from the depths of memory and to celebrate them.

I wish I'd been able to meet Josie. Indeed, I have periodically found myself trying to conjure mental images of his appearance since no photographs from those old days are available. I try to picture his thinning hair and slight stature and somewhat effeminate mannerisms. But even while these physical characteristics remain only vaguely imagined, I truly feel that I have come to know much about Josie through Francis' remembrances. Josie was a mentor to a teenage boy starting to learn carpentry, a middle-aged carpenter with some renown because of an uncanny ability to sharpen saws, and a somewhat eccentric old man who seemed to believe one could never measure and re-measure too many times. Josie was the spirit of an era now receding. And, in a sense, he remains part of our family as we chuckle at his foibles and repeat his favorite aphorisms about carpentry.

To remember Josie is to celebrate the influences that help shape all human lives. Caregivers should be alert to such influences when patients relate their stories. Invariably our appreciation of the human condition is enhanced by attentiveness to the specifics of narrative. To acknowledge important influences is to share in the depth and complexity of human interaction.

References
[1] Bellow S. The Adventures of Augie March. New York: Penguin Books; 1953.

Take Courage

The stories we share with one another are enlightening. They permit a glimpse, and sometimes an immersion, into the hopes and fears, the love and grief that characterize our shared humanity.

Some time ago, a friend recalled the months she spent in London after college. This was a difficult and trying time for Teri. One day, while riding on a commuter train and feeling particularly low, she looked up and saw a large sign that said "Take Courage." It was almost as if this was a personal message directed at her. Teri recalls feeling resolve and determination to carry on. On subsequent days she specifically looked for her sign with its heartening admonition. She recalls that this billboard message truly did help her get through a difficult period in her life. Much later, she realized that the sign was actually an advertisement for a beer called *Courage*. This ironic twist serves to emphasize the poignancy of her account and the veracity of her recollection.

Another friend offered more whimsical reflections. At a recent party, Carl ruefully acknowledged some of his own past idiosyncrasies. He recalled that as a young boy in St. Paul, he spent an entire afternoon on Lexington Avenue shifting two pieces of cardboard under his feet so that he never touched the ground. When this revelation prompted hearty laughter from the assembled guests, this storyteller further acknowledged that in his youth he had another unusual ritual. Upon flushing the upstairs toilet, he would race to the bottom of the stairs in order to reach the ground floor before the toilet ceased running. Carl did not reveal to our gathering what finally led him to break this habit. However, he did share with us another ritual that developed as an adult. His father was gravely ill, thought possibly to be near death. Carl prayed earnestly that his father would survive long enough to take Carl's young son fishing one more time. After his father eventually recovered, Carl recalls going to great lengths to find excuses to keep his son from actually going on a fishing outing with his father. At

141

some level, Carl believed that God had agreed to permit the grandfather and grandson to have one more fishing adventure together. He wanted to defer accepting this gift as far into the future as possible. Carl recalls a summer day when he returned home and discovered that the grandfather had unexpectedly picked up his grandson to do some fishing. When I jokingly asked Carl what happened to his father after this outing, he indicated that "he died," although not for many months thereafter.

Still another friend and academic colleague acknowledges that in his youth he also made a bargain with God. Ron was ten years old when his cousin died of a ruptured appendix. He remembers being fearful and praying that God preserve his life until he was very old. He impulsively chose age 50. As Ron approached his 50th birthday, he began to develop a series of health problems. He also commenced to feel uneasiness about the bargain he had made in his youth. In a narrative entitled "Joining the Majority," Ron offers reflections on death, starting with the Faustian bargain he made as a child and moving to more seasoned perspectives gained by advancing age and experience.[1]

Recently, I unexpectedly found a store that sold *Courage* beer and sampled it for the first time. As I savored the beer, I reflected on a young woman in England finding the inner courage to battle the forces that distressed her. I mused about a loving father employing magical thinking to try to ensure that his son would have more time to spend with his grandfather. And I recalled a middle-aged friend who began to feel the pangs of aging and mortality.

Of course all of these issues and more are part of every clinical practice. It takes courage to cope with the treacheries before us and those that may come.

References

[1] Robinson R. Joining the Majority. In: Olsen A. et al, editors. The Call to Care. Sioux Falls: Ex Machina; 1999.

Sheds

Before pasqueflowers and trillium, before hints of new greenery, the shed antlers appear. They are perched in various attitudes. Sometimes they seem to have come out of the ground itself. The search for deer sheds anticipates spring, but precedes it by weeks. Last year the search began on the first weekend of March. The temperature had climbed into the low 40s but the wind was sharp. We were grateful for our winter garb.

Although Mary and I started the search walking side by side, our paths soon diverged. The business of looking for sheds quickly becomes a contest. At one point, I stood in the vicinity of a new specimen and pretended not to see it as Mary walked up to me. She exclaimed at the prize but was not fooled by my seeming inattention. That day, I quickly found another antler and then a third. Mary sprang back into contention by coming upon a very large specimen, perhaps ruefully dropped by a dominant buck reduced to wondering how he'd keep order absent his crown. As the afternoon wound down, I crossed by the garden. I was getting so close to the house that I did not really expect to find any additional bounty. But as a magnificent conclusion to the afternoon of tramping around the land, I discovered a matched set of antlers at the base of an ash tree. It is uncommon for a deer to drop both antlers at the same time. I believe this was the third occasion in the last five years that someone on our land has found a matched pair of antlers lying together.

My father-in-law, Francis, visited during a shed season. At breakfast, several of us were talking excitedly about the antlers we had found in the preceding days. Francis did not evidence much interest. Later that morning, as he and I were climbing a steep hill in our '49 Jeep, Francis suddenly called out for me to stop. He leaped out of the Jeep and hurried off the trail some ten feet or so to seize a magnificent shed. After that, his enthusiasm was ignited and he spent the next hour roaming across the prairie in search of additional sheds. Such is the nature of shed obsession.

Inevitably, when the yearly ritual of looking for sheds begins, my wife and I find ourselves thinking about Suzanne. She spent the last year of her life in hospice. She had suffered the ravages of juvenile onset diabetes and had sustained multiple strokes. However, Suzanne remained very engaged by ideas and the people around her, and was fascinated by our enthusiastic search for sheds. We presented one to her as a gift and she proudly kept it on her bedside table along with the poem that follows. She seemed quite pleased that I dedicated the piece to her.

Searching for Shed Antlers in March
for Suzanne

When the dull morning became sunshine
on snow, we headed out in search of antlers
shed by deer too preoccupied to sense their loss.
Trails wandered through trees, converging
at times before veering off over another hill.
Scat lent dark accent to furrows of snow
and crisscrossed patches of exposed ground
on south facing slopes. Newly uncovered prairie
lay brittle and brown, exhausted by the winter.

We exclaimed each time another antler was found,
eagerly counting points and our good fortune.
Someone asked how the deer, having lost its crown,
becomes whole again. Much occurs behind our backs.

Good things can follow loss, like insight and expectation.
A new season unfolds. Soon we'll seek pasqueflowers
hidden among the hopeful grasses of spring. [1]

Certainly those of us in health care learn critical data about our patients by carefully listening to their story. Experts, like

Rita Charon, note that caregivers also can learn much through the process of writing. [2] I believe that this poem can serve as a metaphor for clinical work. In particular I like the notion that "much occurs behind our backs," and the hopeful belief that even with serious illness "good things can follow loss."

While looking for sheds is an activity far removed from the domain of illness, this annual ritual shares some commonalities with the work of patient care. Physicians diligently search for remedies for patients' woes. Often, careful clinical analysis yields the desired result. On occasion, serendipity and good fortune may assist diagnostic acumen. At times, when a curative intervention is not possible, our mere presence and concern may be a balm. Our willingness to figuratively walk with the patient in search of respite may resemble those times when we eagerly traipse across the prairie but fail to find sheds. Surely our efforts are worthwhile even when the goal remains elusive. There is solace in the commitment to press forward.

References
[1] Freeman J. Searching for Shed Antlers in March. South Dakota Magazine. 2005 March/April.
[2] Charon, R. Narrative and medicine. New England Journal of Medicine. 2004 February 26: 350: 862-4.

What Are Those Doctors Saying?

A Glossary for Laypersons

(Editor's Note: Doctors and other professionals don't use jargon to confuse us ordinary folks. It's just that technical terms stand for particular ideas that are often difficult to explain in plain English. In fact, many ordinary words do the same thing. Imagine trying to talk about the moon, for example, without using the word "moon." As long as we agree on the meaning of a word, it can be used as a kind of shortcut expressing sometimes complicated, yet quite precise, ideas. Doctors have taken a long time learning the code words of their profession, and when they talk with each other they speak quite efficiently and with confidence that they are understood. A non-doctor listening in, however, may be bewildered by what sounds like gobbledygook. Since the essays in this book were originally written by a doctor for other doctors, some of those technical medical terms were used. In this glossary, we picked some of the words relating to medicine and bioethics that may give a layperson trouble and have tried to define them in the simplest, non-technical way we know how. — R.L.R.)

The four bioethical principles:

Autonomy — Respect for individuals and their ability to make decisions about their own health. Leaving the patient out of the decision-making process is to be avoided.
Beneficence — Decisions intended to benefit the patient.
Non-maleficence — Decisions intended to do no harm to the patient.
Justice — Decisions intended to be fair, not only to the patient, but also to others who may be involved.

146

Medical Terms (and some others, as well):

Ankylosing Spondylitis — inflammation of the spine and large joints resulting in pain, stiffness and severe loss of mobility.

Aphasia — Loss of the ability to understand and/or express ideas in language due to an injury to the brain.

Aplastic Anemia — A deficiency in the oxygen-carrying ability of blood caused by the underproduction of red blood cells in the bone marrow.

CAT — (Computed Axial Tomography) An x-ray technique that shows the brain and other parts of the body in serial slices.

Colostrum — The fluid, rich in antibodies and minerals, that exudes from the mammary glands just before the production of true milk after a female gives birth.

DNA — (DeoxiriboNucleic Acid) The chain of chemicals, often referred to as "the double helix," which carries genetic information determining bodily characteristics passed along by heredity.

DRG — (Diagnosis-Related Group) A Medicare formula for reimbursing hospitals based on disease type and treatment required.

EEG — (Electroencephalogram) The electric activity of the brain as recorded on a graph, used in diagnosing brain disorders.

Endoscopic — Related to the endoscope, an instrument used to look at the interior organs of the body.

Endarterectomy — Surgical removal of blockage of artery constricted by fatty deposits.

Etiology — The study of the origins or causes of diseases.

Gastroenterology — The study of disorders affecting the stomach, intestines, and related organs.

Glioblastoma — A malignant tumor of the brain..

H-pylori — (Helicobacter pylori) Bacteria that can cause ulcers and inflammation of the stomach.

Hematologic — Relating to the study of blood.

Hepatic — Relating to the liver.

147

Hyperbaric Oxygen — Oxygen delivered under pressure higher than normal atmospheric pressure.

Lapstrake — In boatbuilding, hull made with overlapping planks.

MRI — (Magnetic Resonance Imaging) A technique that uses a powerful magnetic field to align the nuclei of cells in order to generate detailed images of the brain and other parts of the body.

Myelin — A white, fatty covering of some nerve fibers.

Paradigm — A model or pattern.

Postural hypotension — Fall in blood pressure that results from going from a reclining or seated position to a standing position: head rush.

Psychogenic — Originating in the mind or by mental/emotional processes, rather than from some other physical disease state.

Organicity — A physical disease in some body organ.

Otitis media — Infection of the middle ear, often causing pain and loss of hearing.

Recombinant DNA — DNA prepared by transplantation into an organism of a different species. It may then be replicated.

Somatoform — Applied to situations in which a patient shows symptoms that cannot be linked to physical causes. The symptoms may cause actual pain and distress, but no connection can be made to an anatomic disease state.

T-lymphocytes — A form of white blood cell that helps protect against viral infections and some forms of cancer cells.

Thoracic — Related to the chest, or thorax.

Thrombosis — Obstruction of an artery or a vein by a blood clot.

About the Author

Jerome W. Freeman, M.D., is a practicing physician and educator. He is on the faculties of the University of South Dakota School of Medicine and of Augustana College. He has a particular interest in biomedical ethics and the use of literature for teaching about illness, the patient, and the caregiver. His previous publications include three books of poetry, *Something at Last* (1993), *Easing the Edges* (1994) and *Starting from Here* (1996), a book of essays *Come and See* (1995), as well as sections in *The Call To Care* (1999).